AJPH

A PUBLICATION OF THE
AMERICAN PUBLIC HEALTH ASSOCIATION

AMERICAN JOURNAL of PUBLIC HEALTH
MARCH 2023
Issue 3

US PUBLIC HEALTH LAW IN THE AFTERMATH OF COVID-19

Challenges, p. 267
Judicial Review of Public Health Powers, pp. 272 and 280
State Public Health Emergency Laws, pp. 275 and 288
The 2023 Supreme Court, p. 269

Also in this issue:

ADOLESCENT HEALTH
Economic Empowerment and HIV, pp. 246 and 306
Our Future, p. 249

REPRODUCTIVE RIGHTS
Parental Consent for Abortion, p. 316

RELATIONSHIP VIOLENCE
School-Based Interventions, p. 320
Related to Pregnancy, p. 297

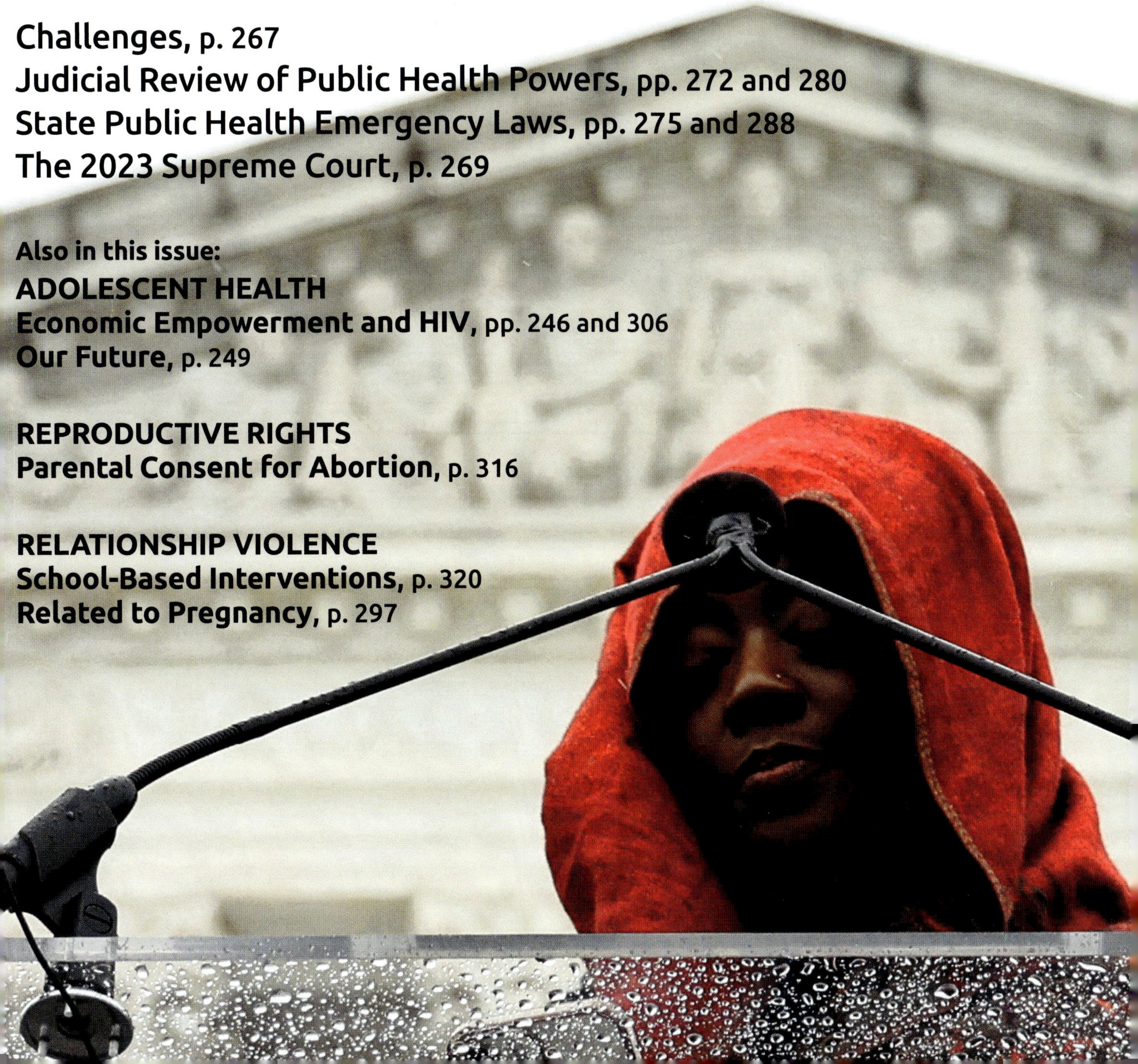

APHA
AMERICAN PUBLIC HEALTH ASSOCIATION
For science. For action. For health.

AJPH®, published monthly, is the official Journal of the American Public Health Association®, 800 I St NW, Washington, DC 20001-3710; (202) 777- APHA; TDD (202) 777-2500. APHA is a nongovernmental professional society founded in 1872, representing all disciplines and specialties in public health.

The *American Journal of Public Health*® (*AJPH*) (print ISSN: 0090-0036; electronic ISSN: 1541- 0048), first published in 1911, is the official journal of the American Public Health Association® (APHA). The oldest and largest organization of public health professionals in the world, APHA represents approximately 30 000 members from more than 50 occupations of public health.

Submissions: Visit www.editorialmanager.com/ajph or ajph.edmgr.com for online manuscript preparation and submission guidelines. Contributions of original unpublished research, social science analyses, scholarly essays, critical commentaries, departments, and letters to the editor are welcome. Questions? Write ajph.submissions@apha.org or call APHA at (202) 777-2469.

Print plus online subscriptions: Institutional price (print copy with online access for a single institution and all authorized users, regardless of geographic location) varies by size of organization and ranges from $993–$1445 for US organizations, and $1073–$1526 for international organizations (air delivery); multiple campuses not permitted without special arrangement. Details of the tiered pricing system at https://subscriptionoffice.com/pages/apha-landing-page. To order, write apha.subscriptions@apha.org.

Online only subscriptions: Institutional price for one institution and its authorized users (regardless of geographic location) is $878–$1307. To order, write apha.subscriptions@apha.org. For academic consortia or multisite corporate subscriptions, contact apha.subscriptions@apha.org.

Print-only subscriptions: Institutional price is US $701, $782 international.

Back print issues: A limited number of print issues are for sale. Single copies are US $49, $55 international (air delivery). Shipping included; prepay only. To order, write apha.subscriptions@apha.org.

Reprints: For prices and ordering information on 50 or more reprints, check the Reprints section at www.ajph.org. To order smaller quantities of reprints (rush delivery), use the "Purchase Article" link on the article site itself.

Electronic access: Online articles more than 10 years old are available free for personal use at www.ajph.org. Recent articles are available through pay-per-view: single PDF article for $24, single issue access for 24 hours for $33, or entire site access for 24 hours for $38.

Postal information: Periodicals postage paid at Washington, DC, and additional mailing offices. Postmaster: Send address changes to American Journal of Public Health, 800 I St NW, Washington, DC 20001-3710.

Address changes: Send to AJPH, Membership Department (members) or AJPH Subscriptions (subscribers), APHA, 800 I St NW, Washington, DC 20001-3710. Or write to membership.mail@apha. org (members) or apha.subscriptions@apha.org (subscribers).

Advertising: For pricing and other information, see www.ajph.org. Please write to ashell.alston@apha.org or call (202) 777-2470 for other advertising opportunities. Ask about special exhibit packages and sponsorships. Acceptance of advertising by the *Journal* does not imply endorsement of products.

Indexes: Publications that index or abstract articles from AJPH include the following: Ageline, Assia (Applied Social Science Index and Abstracts), Biological Abstracts, Chemical Abstracts, CINAHL, Criminal Justice Abstracts, EMBASE, EMCare, Environmental Abstracts, e-psyche, ERIC, ETOH (Alcohol and Alcohol Problems Science Database), Excerpta Medica, Food Science and Technology, General Science Index, Grateful Med, Hospital Literature Index, Human Resources Abstracts, International Pharmaceutical Abstracts (IPA), Medline, Physical Education Index, Pollution Abstracts, Psychological Abstracts, PsychINFO, Safety Science Abstracts, Sage Family Studies Abstracts, Sage Human Resources Abstracts, Science Citation Index, SCOPUS, SIIC Data Bases, Social Work Research and Abstracts, and Statistical Reference Index (SRI)/LexisNexis.

Medscape Publishers' Circle

AJPH

A PUBLICATION OF THE
AMERICAN PUBLIC HEALTH ASSOCIATION

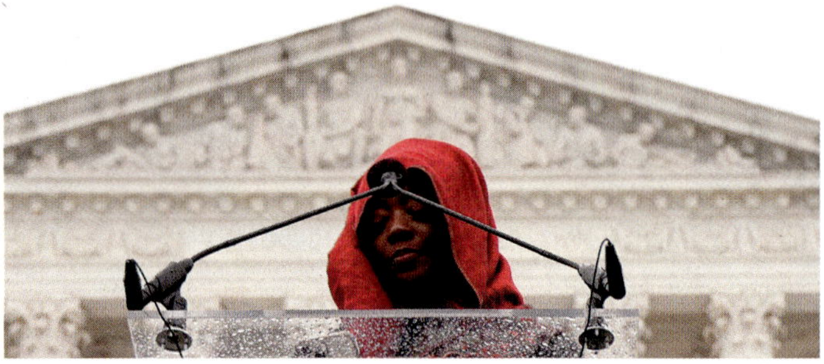

COVER: Michelle Mabson, co-founder of Black Millennials 4 Flint, joins fellow environmental activists gathering outside as the US Supreme Court hears arguments in *Sackett v. EPA*, which could limit the scope of the federal landmark Clean Water Act of 1972, on the first day of the court's new term in Washington, DC, October 3, 2022.

Cover concept and selection by Aleisha Kropf. Photo by REUTERS/ Jonathan Ernst. Printed with permission.

APHA
AMERICAN PUBLIC HEALTH ASSOCIATION
For science. For action. For health.

Promoting public health research, policy, practice, and education is the *AJPH* mission. As we widen our scope to embrace global issues, we also sharpen our focus to support the needs of public health practitioners. We invite contributions of original unpublished research, opinion and commentary, and letters to the editor.

The *Journal* is printed on acid-free recycled paper.

OPEN ACCESS | ONLINE ONLY | PODCAST | DATA SUPPLEMENT AVAILABLE

EDITOR'S CHOICE

245 Publishing in the *American Journal of Public Health*: Don't Be Desk Rejected
A. Morabia and M. C. Costanza

OPINIONS, IDEAS, & PRACTICE

EDITORIALS

246 Multilevel Interventions to Improve Adolescent Mental Health in Low- and Middle-Income Countries
S. E. Baumann and B. Devkota

249 Protecting and Promoting Adolescent Health: A Public Health of Consequence, March 2023
F. Kapadia

PERSPECTIVES

251 Caring for Military-Affiliated Transgender and Gender-Diverse Youths: A Call for Protections
D. A. Klein, N. A. Schvey, T. A. Baxter, N. S. Larson, and C. M. Roberts

256 The Future of Pharmacist-Delivered Status-Neutral HIV Prevention and Care
P. J. Weidle, J. T. Brooks, S.S. Valentine, and D. Daskalakis

259 Is the Goal of "The Healthiest Nation" Attainable or Desirable?
N. Zohoori

262 Achieving Healthiest Nation Status Is Both Attainable and Desirable
G. C. Benjamin

NOTES FROM THE FIELD

263 A Community-Engaged Social Marketing Campaign to Promote Equitable Access to COVID-19 Services Among Latino Immigrants
H. S. Shah, A. F. Miller, C. Yang, S. M. Grieb, M. Lipke, B. F. Bigelow, K. H. Phillips, P. Palomino, and K. R. Page

CHALLENGES TO PUBLIC HEALTH LAW IN THE AFTERMATH OF COVID-19

267 The Challenges to Public Health Law in the Aftermath of COVID-19
W. E. Parmet and P. C. Erwin

269 The 2023 US Supreme Court Term: Implications for Public Health
L. F. Wiley

272 Judicial Trends in the Era of COVID-19: Public Health in Peril
L. O. Gostin

275 State Public Health Emergency Powers in Response to COVID-19
J. G. Hodge Jr., L. T. Dunning, and J. L. Piatt

RESEARCH & ANALYSIS

CHALLENGES TO PUBLIC HEALTH LAW IN THE AFTERMATH OF COVID-19

280 Judicial Review of Public Health Powers Since the Start of the COVID-19 Pandemic: Trends and Implications
W. E. Parmet and F. Khalik

288 Trends in US State Public Health Emergency Laws, 2021–2022
E. Platt, K. Moran-McCabe, A. Cook, and S. Burris

PERSPECTIVES FROM THE SOCIAL SCIENCES

297 Screening for and Experiences of Intimate Partner Violence in the United States Before, During, and After Pregnancy, 2016–2019
K. B. Kozhimannil, V. A. Lewis, J. D. Interrante, P. L. Chastain, and L. Admon

SURVEILLANCE

306 Economic Empowerment, HIV Risk Behavior, and Mental Health Among School-Going Adolescent Girls in Uganda: Longitudinal Cluster-Randomized Controlled Trial, 2017–2022
F. M. Ssewamala, R. Brathwaite, and T. B. Neilands

OPEN-THEMED RESEARCH

316 Use of Judicial Bypass of Mandatory Parental Consent to Access Abortion and Judicial Bypass Denials, Florida and Texas, 2018–2021
A. J. Stevenson and K. Coleman-Minahan

320 School-Based Interventions to Prevent Dating and Relationship Violence and Gender-Based Violence: Systematic Review and Network Meta-Analysis
C. Farmer, N. Shaw, A. J. Rizzo, N. Orr, A. Chollet, A. Hagell, E. Rigby, H. Young, V. Berry, C. Bonell, and G. J. Melendez-Torres

331 Dollar Stores and Food Access for Rural Households in the United States, 2008–2020
W. Feng, E. T. Page, and S. B. Cash

BACKMATTER

OTHER DEPARTMENTS

337 Career Opportunities

344 Subscription Form

LETTERS & RESPONSES

e1 Breast Cancer Prevention Misinformation on Pinterest: One Side of a Thick Coin
S. M. Modell, A. H. Ponte, H. R. Director, S. K. Pettersen, S. L. R. Kardia, and H. H. Goltz

e2 Wilner and Holton Respond
T. Wilner and A. Holton

ERRATA

e4 Erratum In: "The Cruel Public Health Consequences of Anti-Immigrant Rhetoric"

Publishing in the *American Journal of Public Health*: Don't Be Desk Rejected

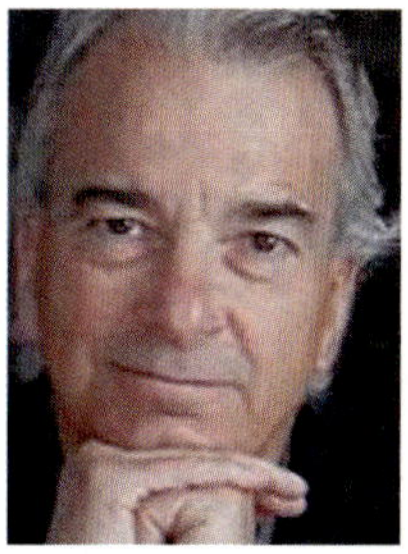

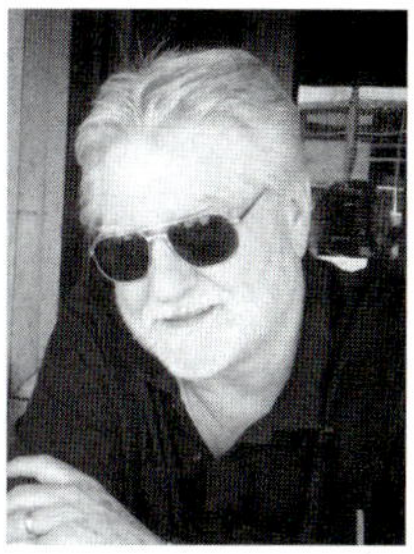

Since June 2015, we have received about 30 000 submissions. We have enjoyed many of them, but we also have learned quite a bit about our prospective authors' submission approaches.

Here is how our review process is organized: All submissions are first triaged by the editor-in-chief and the senior deputy editor. Out of 100 new submissions, 33% are internally "desk rejected" (i.e., without further review), sometimes without being deeply read, because their content is not appropriate for this journal. This has nothing to do with their quality. If their content is appropriate, some common causes of desk rejection are outdated data (e.g., data collection completed > 3 years before [which is too old for *AJPH*]); analysis of surveys not based on the latest data release; results of primarily etiological interest; pilot, feasibility, formative or process evaluation, or validation studies; lack of a comparison or control group; low survey response rate(s); small samples; case studies; and convenience samples. Of the 67% left, another half are desk rejected because they are deemed to be of low priority in terms of novelty or mainly of local interest—the *Journal* favoring national data when it comes to surveys and surveillance.

The 33% of submissions retained beyond the triage stage are forwarded to the deputy editor, who decides whether to assign them to an associate editor. A substantial number of rejections "without reviews" occur at this stage. Beyond it, the papers either will be rejected "after review" or published.

These statistics are for all submissions, including Opinion Pieces and Notes From the Field. If we focus specifically on Research Articles, Brief Research Articles, Analytic Essays, and Public Health Then and Now history manuscripts, which are strictly externally peer-reviewed, a simple way to put it is that 90% are rejected without review. We are very selective but make a huge effort to process these articles quickly. Five percent will be rejected after review, and 5% will be published. Both outcomes should be considered as successful, because the external reviews mean that peers have been working on your paper, and their comments may help you in publishing the paper elsewhere. The problem is the 90% of desk rejections, which involve a large loss of time and are a source of unwarranted frustration.

These desk rejections can be dramatically reduced if one reads the Instructions for Authors carefully and familiarizes oneself with the mission of *AJPH* by perusing its tables of contents over a few months and reading the most relevant articles. Explaining in the cover letter what the paper adds to what the *Journal* has already published is also useful. At triage, we are not necessarily aware of the whole literature, but we are aware of what we have published.

Targeting the submission to a journal that is expecting similar articles may be time consuming, but it is worth allocating sufficient time to this search given that getting funded, conducting the research, and preparing the paper may have taken years.

As a bottom line, desk-rejected articles are as frustrating for us as they are for you. A useful objective is to carefully target a journal in order primarily not to be desk rejected because, again, having external reviews increases the chances of an article being published quickly and well, whereas a desk rejection just leaves the same paper older.

We feel that the knowledge we have today after triaging 30 000 submissions would have been useful when we were researchers aspiring to publish, but, hopefully, these comments may be of great interest for young researchers or researchers coming from institutions where specific training about how to publish quickly and well is neglected. AJPH

Alfredo Morabia, MD, PhD
Editor-in-Chief
AJPH
Michael C. Costanza, PhD
Senior Deputy Editor
AJPH

DOI: https://doi.org/10.2105/AJPH.2022.307218

55 Years Ago

Abortion Law: The Approaches of Different Nations

In the United States, the estimated one to one and a half million criminal abortions that occur each year cause much more extensive damage than the few hundred recorded deaths would indicate. It is estimated that 350,000 women a year suffer postoperative complications from abortion. . . . The difficulty in coping with this disastrous situation is that abortion is not solely a medical problem. . . . In those jurisdictions in which the law makes it a crime to perform an abortion except to save the life of the woman, the physician's hands are tied. . . . The stringency of such laws drives women to self-inflicted abortions, to abortions performed by unqualified persons, and to abortions performed by qualified persons under improper conditions. . . . Periodic repression of "abortion rings" and prosecution of individual physicians, however, have failed utterly to halt the resort of desperate women (the majority of whom are married) to criminal abortionists. . . . As the history of prohibition indicates, a law which attempts to legislate morals and which does not have the support of the people is unenforceable.

From AJPH, November 1967, pp. 1906–1907

82 Years Ago

Public Health and the Law

Practitioners of public health should bear in mind that the police power under which they conduct their functions is broad in scope, is usually construed liberally by the courts, and always gives them ample authority for their operations, but they must also remember that there are limitations upon the police power imposed by constitutions and the common law. Under our form of government, citizens have certain inalienable rights which the courts are zealous to safeguard.

From AJPH, June 1941, p. 591

Multilevel Interventions to Improve Adolescent Mental Health in Low- and Middle-Income Countries

Sara E. Baumann, PhD, MPH, and Bhimsen Devkota, PhD

ABOUT THE AUTHORS

Sara E. Baumann is with the Department of Behavioral and Community Health Sciences, School of Public Health, University of Pittsburgh, Pittsburgh, PA. Bhimsen Devkota is with the Department of Health Education, Faculty of Education, Tribhuvan University, Kirtipur, Nepal.

See also Ssewamala et al., p. 306.

AJPH March 2023, Vol 113, No. 3

Adolescence is a formative period in which foundational social and emotional habits are shaped, which inform health and well-being throughout the life course. It is a time of pronounced transition—physiologically, socially, and emotionally. Several lifelong risk factors put children and adolescents at risk for mental disorders, including but not limited to nutritional status; caregivers' physical and mental health; exposure to violence, armed conflict, and war; natural disasters; and gender disparities.[1] When one or more of these factors coalesce, adolescents become vulnerable to poor mental health outcomes.[2] Globally, one in seven adolescents experiences mental health conditions, which often go undiagnosed and untreated.[3] This is of urgent concern in low- and middle-income countries (LMICs), where resources to detect and treat mental health concerns among children and adolescents are limited.[1]

RISK-TAKING BEHAVIOR AND MENTAL HEALTH

Poor mental health has broad-reaching effects, in both the immediate and the long term. Directly relevant to the findings of Ssewamala et al., published in this issue of *AJPH* (p. 306), is the link between mental health and HIV risk-taking behavior. Specifically, poor mental health conditions can lead to increased risk-taking behavior, including early sexual activity, resulting in higher risk for HIV and other sexually transmitted infections and unwanted pregnancy.[1] Youths often seek out risk-taking behaviors to cope with emotional difficulties. For example, research by Brown et al. highlights that adolescents with a major depressive disorder struggle with self-esteem and assertiveness, which are critical for supporting safer sex practices.[4] Therefore, providing youths with appropriate and safe coping mechanisms and skills to regulate emotions and build resilience for overcoming adversity is needed to improve youths' mental health, reproductive health, and other health concerns.[2]

ECONOMIC EMPOWERMENT AND MENTAL HEALTH

In LMICs, poverty can have detrimental effects on social and emotional development in children.[5] Financial insecurity directly affects life decisions at the household level, which in turn affect health. Often, limited household income puts parents under pressure to choose between meeting the needs of sons versus the needs of daughters. Preference for sons over daughters is widespread globally, particularly in Asia and North Africa. A review of data from 66 developing countries found that preference given to sons disproportionally affects children of disadvantaged backgrounds, such as rural and poor families.[6] As a result of prioritizing sons' needs, daughters tend to experience poorer health and development outcomes, such as malnutrition and dropping out of school, where they could have gained critical information about sexual health, HIV, and other health issues as well as the interpersonal and communication skills needed to negotiate in health decision-making. Out-of-school girls are also more likely to engage in risk-taking activities, such as transactional and unprotected sex, to either meet immediate financial needs or increase their social and economic status.[7]

To address these risks, conditional cash transfers are an example of a programmatic approach that seeks to improve financial security and, in doing so, can improve health and education outcomes. Such programs provide cash to families if they follow certain requirements, which allows families to meet immediate household needs and encourages them to invest in their children's health and development.[8] Oportunidades, implemented in Mexico, is one of the first conditional cash transfer programs and serves as a global model.[9] Cash is provided to the female head of household, conditional on children attending school and the family taking part in preventive health education talks. A randomized control trial of

Oportunidades demonstrated reduced socioemotional problems in children aged 8 to 10 years and reduced behavioral problems. Thus, receiving cash reduces economic stress on the household and improves parental mental health and family relationships, directly affecting the mental health outcomes of children and adolescents.[9] Furthermore, a systematic review by Klasen and Crombag indicates that parental training and engagement is promising for addressing behavioral disorders in LMICs.[10]

INTERVENTION

Acknowledging the importance of economic security is the foundation for the intervention of Ssewamala et al., which aims to reduce HIV risk-taking and improve mental health in Uganda. The authors investigated the effect of an economic empowerment intervention on HIV risk behaviors and mental health among school-going adolescent girls. Although the intervention did not have significant effects on HIV risk behaviors, likely because of the young age of the participants, it significantly improved mental health outcomes for participants. This work, importantly, provides a model that combines an economic intervention with family strengthening, which can be applied in LMIC contexts to improve youth mental health.

Ssewamala et al. tested two arms of the intervention. The first was Youth Development Accounts (YDAs), in which each participant was provided a savings account with matched one-to-one funding. The second arm of the intervention included YDAs plus Multiple Family Group, a 16-session intervention facilitated by parents and community health workers that aimed to strengthen family relationships. The Multiple Family Group sessions included children, caregivers, siblings, and extended family members such as aunts, uncles, and grandparents. Training addressed an array of topics, including health knowledge and behaviors, stigma and discrimination, building family strengths, problem-solving at home, and respectful communication.

To test the intervention, participants were randomized at the school level to one of three options: (1) standard health and sex education (control), (2) YDA, and (3) YDA plus Multiple Family Group. Although both interventions that went beyond the standard health and sex education witnessed significantly lower depressive symptoms and better self-concept among participants, the YDA plus Multiple Family Group participants had significantly lower hopelessness than did those in the control group. This suggests that an economic intervention combined with family strengthening is a promising approach for improving mental health among adolescent girls.

LEVELS OF THE SOCIOECOLOGICAL MODEL

The work of Ssewamala et al. establishes the importance of intervening at multiple levels of the socioecological model for maximum impact. For example, in the Uganda study, intervening at the individual level through YDAs significantly improved mental health; however, the intervention that included an additional component of family strengthening (i.e., interpersonal level) had a positive impact on hopelessness, which was not found in the YDA arm of the intervention. These findings suggest that adolescent mental health is influenced by a variety of factors and that improving family life in combination with economic security can significantly affect mental health outcomes and outlook on life.

Future interventions aiming to build on this work may consider multilevel interventions that intervene not only at the individual and family level but also at the organizational, community, and policy levels. One example of this is intervention through peer education at school as part of the national curriculum. Another approach is intervention through women's groups and microfinance groups at the community level, which have demonstrated promise for addressing other complex health issues among youths such as malnutrition and child marriage.[11,12] Finally, establishing a supportive policy environment that protects the rights of youths—such as child marriage laws—will help to ensure a fruitful living environment for healthy decision-making and improved health.

CONCLUSIONS

The findings of Ssewamala et al. highlight the importance of intervening at multiple levels. The intervention illuminates the critical link between economic status, family functioning, and mental health outcomes, which demonstrates potential for future scaling to improve adolescent health in LMICs. AJPH

CORRESPONDENCE

Correspondence should be sent to Sara E. Baumann, 130 DeSoto St, Pittsburgh, PA 15261 (e-mail: sarabaumann@pitt.edu). Reprints can be ordered at http://www.ajph.org by clicking the "Reprints" link.

PUBLICATION INFORMATION

Full Citation: Baumann SE, Devkota B. Multilevel interventions to improve adolescent mental health in low- and middle-income countries. *Am J Public Health*. 2023;113(3):246–248.

Acceptance Date: December 12, 2022.

DOI: https://doi.org/10.2105/AJPH.2022.307201

CONTRIBUTORS

S. E. Baumann led the writing of the editorial. B. Devkota reviewed and edited the editorial.

CONFLICTS OF INTEREST

The authors have no conflicts of interest to declare.

REFERENCES

1. Kieling C, Baker-Henningham H, Belfer M, et al. Child and adolescent mental health worldwide: evidence for action. *Lancet.* 2011;378(9801): 1515–1525. https://doi.org/10.1016/S0140-6736(11)60827-1
2. World Health Organization. Adolescent mental health. Available at: https://www.who.int/news-room/fact-sheets/detail/adolescent-mental-health. Accessed December 19, 2022.
3. Institute for Health Metrics and Evaluation. Global Burden of Disease Study. Available at: https://www.healthdata.org/gbd/2019. Accessed December 19, 2022.
4. Brown LK, Danovsky MB, Lourie KJ, DiClemente RJ, Ponton LE. Adolescents with psychiatric disorders and the risk of HIV. *J Am Acad Child Adolesc Psychiatry.* 1997;36(11):1609–1617. https://doi.org/10.1016/S0890-8567(09)66573-4
5. Grantham-McGregor S, Cheung YB, Cueto S, et al.; International Child Development Steering Group. Developmental potential in the first 5 years for children in developing countries. *Lancet.* 2007; 369(9555):60–70. https://doi.org/10.1016/S0140-6736(07)60032-4
6. Le K, Nguyen M. Son preference and health disparities in developing countries. *SSM Popul Health.* 2022;17:101036. https://doi.org/10.1016/j.ssmph.2022.101036
7. Luke N, Kurz K. Cross-generational and transactional sexual relations in Sub-Saharan Africa. 2002. Available at: https://www.icrw.org/wp-content/uploads/2016/10/Cross-generational-and-Transactional-Sexual-Relations-in-Sub-Saharan-Africa-Prevalence-of-Behavior-and-Implications-for-Negotiating-Safer-Sexual-Practices.pdf. Accessed December 9, 2022.
8. de Janvry A, Sadoulet E. Making conditional cash transfer programs more efficient: designing for maximum effect of the conditionality. *World Bank Econ Rev.* 2006;20(1):1–29. https://doi.org/10.1093/wber/lhj002
9. Fernald LC, Gertler PJ, Neufeld LM. 10-year effect of Oportunidades, Mexico's conditional cash transfer programme, on child growth, cognition, language, and behaviour: a longitudinal follow-up study. *Lancet.* 2009;374(9706):1997–2005. [Erratum in: *Lancet.* 2010;376(9755):1828]. https://doi.org/10.1016/S0140-6736(09)61676-7
10. Klasen H, Crombag AC. What works where? A systematic review of child and adolescent mental health interventions for low and middle income countries. *Soc Psychiatry Psychiatr Epidemiol.* 2013; 48(4):595–611. https://doi.org/10.1007/s00127-012-0566-x
11. Amigó MF, Gurung S. The transformational possibilities of a peer education program to address child marriage in Nepal. *Dev Pract.* 2022;32(7): 890–900. https://doi.org/10.1080/09614524.2021.1937572
12. Upreti YR, Bastien S, Bjønness B, Devkota B. The socio-ecological model as a framework for understanding junk food consumption among schoolchildren in Nepal. *Nutr Health.* 2021;27(3): 337–346. https://doi.org/10.1177/02601060211000169

Protecting and Promoting Adolescent Health: A Public Health of Consequence, March 2023

Farzana Kapadia, PhD, MPH

ABOUT THE AUTHOR

Farzana Kapadia is the deputy editor of AJPH *and a professor of epidemiology at the School of Global Public Health, New York University, NY.*

This issue of *AJPH* presents information on interventions and policies related to two critical determinants of adolescent health and well-being: dating- and relationship-based violence and access to abortion care. Adolescence and young adulthood—roughly ages 15 to 24 years—is marked by cognitive, biological, emotional, and psychosocial development. Successful and healthy development across these domains is foundational for transitioning into healthy adulthood. However, widespread inequities in access to quality education, housing and food security, and culturally and developmentally appropriate health care services, as well as living in unsafe family, peer, or neighborhood environments can disrupt healthy development during this period. Additionally, experiences of dating violence or unintended pregnancy and their associated physical and mental health burdens can undermine successful transition into adulthood. Findings presented in this issue of *AJPH* on dating violence prevention and access to abortion care for adolescents can inform future policy and practice to protect adolescent health and well-being and ultimately promote successful transition into healthy adulthood.

PREVENTING ADOLESCENT DATING VIOLENCE

The prevalence of dating and relationship violence (DRV) among adolescents and young adults varies across national surveys and local studies because of differences in methodology, sampling, recruitment, definition of DRV, and fear and stigma associated with disclosure. Despite these differences, one thing is clear: DRV is highly prevalent in the United States. Findings from the Centers for Disease Control and Prevention's 2019 Youth Risk Behavior Survey indicate that 1 in 8 high school students in a relationship in the past year experienced physical violence and that 1 in 12 experienced sexual dating violence. Estimates for both were higher among female as well as lesbian, gay, bisexual, transgender or transexual, and queer (LGBTQ+) high school students. The 2016–2017 National Intimate Partner and Sexual Violence Survey found that 27.1% of female and 21.4% of male respondents experienced sexual or physical violence or stalking by an intimate partner before they were 18 years old.[1] Growing evidence points to cyberdating violence—improper use of social media and technology to harass, control, and abuse dating partners—as having similar harmful effects as in-person dating violence (https://bit.ly/3uYk5vt).

Preventing adolescent dating violence requires effective interventions that can be delivered widely during the preadolescent years. To this end, Farmer et al. (p. 320) conducted a meta-analysis of school-based interventions targeting DRV and gender-based violence (GBV). Included interventions had a stronger impact on reducing DRV than GBV, and intervention influences on attitude and knowledge were short term. Consequently, school-based interventions ought to be considered as one component of a broader range of preventive actions that weaken social acceptance of DRV and GBV.

ENSURING ACCESS TO SAFE ABORTION CARE

In 1979, the US Supreme Court ruled in *Bellotti v. Baird* that a Massachusetts statute requiring minors younger than 18 years to obtain parental consent to have an abortion was unconstitutional. The court held that parents could not have absolute veto power over a minor's decision to have an abortion and that all minors, as long as they were deemed mature and fully competent to make the decision, had a right to seek judicial authorization for an abortion.

Currently, 36 US states mandate parental involvement in the form of parental consent from one or both parents before an abortion can be performed or parental notification by the medical provider 24 to 48 hours before the abortion (https://bit.ly/2HsVlE1). In 35 states where abortion care is still legal but parental involvement is mandated, seeking judicial bypass as ruled in *Bellotti v. Baird* is available but requires overcoming significant

AJPH March 2023, Vol 113, No. 3

hurdles. Most often, these barriers include lack of knowledge of the judicial bypass process and lack of availability of legal support to navigate the judicial system that lead to delays in abortion care seeking, increase associated costs, and limit the type of care available (https://bit.ly/3Qbc5kt).

With the Supreme Court decision in *Dobbs v. Jackson Women's Health Organization* (2022) overturning the landmark decision in *Roe v. Wade* (1973), minors' ability to obtain abortion care significantly worsened. Stevenson and Coleman-Minahan (p. 316) provide data that sheds light on minors who are forced to travel from states that have newly banned abortion care as a result of the *Dobbs* decision to states that do not have such bans but do require the adolescent to obtain judicial bypass of parental involvement. Their findings reveal that Florida denied judicial bypass petitions at higher rates during 2020 to 2021 than in previous years. The harmful short- and long-term socioeconomic[2] and health and well-being outcomes for both adolescents denied judicial bypass and their offspring are well documented (https://bit.ly/3GB8Zn0).

Additionally, Stevenson and Coleman-Minahan offer two key metrics for tracking the burden on minors of parental involvement laws: judicial bypasses granted among minors obtaining an abortion and proportion of bypass denials among all bypasses sought. Providing such information is critical—without it, we lack information and evidence on the population-level burden of parental involvement laws on abortion care among minors. In addition, we lack information on how bypass denials are shaped by subjective judicial opinions on maturity or competence and whether and how these opinions differ for different groups of minors.

PROMOTING A HEALTHY ADOLESCENCE

Shifting the social and cultural norms that enable adolescent dating violence requires family-, community-, and structural-level interventions to bolster the impact of school-based interventions. By moving beyond individual-based interventions, we can shift our attention to policies and practices that change the contexts, structures, and systems that allow acceptance of adolescent dating violence and likely achieve long-term success. For example, equally necessary are intervening in school- and university-based policies on handling DRV and GBV, strengthening the ability of those who have experienced DRV or GBV to take criminal and legal action, providing appropriate counseling services and mental health care, and advocating efforts to support adolescents and young adults who have experienced DRV or GBV.

Additionally, dating violence intervention efforts need to be culturally relevant and appropriate for racially and ethnically diverse youths and LGBTQ+ youths. To achieve this goal, and as described by De La Rue, DRV interventions require an intersectional approach that addresses racial-, gender-, and sexual orientation-based discrimination to address the lived realities that adolescents and young adults navigate to have safe and healthy realtionships.[3]

Protecting the autonomy of minors to determine whether to continue or discontinue a pregnancy, as decided in *Bellotti v Baird*, is in line with the reproductive justice framework. As the landscape of abortion care shifts across the United States, we can look to past programs that have successfully assisted minors seeking confidential abortion care. For example, between 2013 and 2022—when parental involvement was still mandated in Illinois—the American Civil Liberties Union of Illinois operated the Judicial Bypass Coordination Project. Over this period, the project provided a hotline that offered information about the judicial bypass process and free legal support for minors seeking abortion care throughout the state (https://www.aclu-il.org/en/pna).

Comprehensive practices and policies that lessen threats to a healthy adolescence, particularly related to DRV and judicial bypass denials for abortion care, are critical public health actions that allow adolescents to flourish, gain independence, and transition into successful adulthood. Attention to both of these distinct, but related, public health issues promotes health not just for this generation of adolescents but for our future. AJPH

CORRESPONDENCE

Correspondence should be sent to Farzana Kapadia, PhD, MPH, New York University, School of Global Public Health, 708 Broadway, Room 729, New York, NY 10003 (e-mail: farzana.kapadia@nyu.edu). Reprints can be ordered at http://www.ajph.org by clicking the "Reprints" link.

PUBLICATION INFORMATION

Full Citation: Kapadia F. Protecting and promoting adolescent health: a public health of consequence, March 2023. *Am J Public Health*. 2023; 113(3):249–250.

Acceptance Date: December 19, 2022.

DOI: https://doi.org/10.2105/AJPH.2022.307209

CONFLICTS OF INTEREST

The author has no conflicts of interest to disclose.

REFERENCES

1. Leemis RW, Friar N, Khatiwada S, et al. *The National Intimate Partner and Sexual Violence Survey: 2016/2017 Report on Intimate Partner Violence*. Atlanta, GA: National Center for Injury Prevention and Control, Centers for Disease Control and Prevention; 2022.
2. Foster DG, Ralph LJ, Biggs MA, Gerdts C, Roberts SCM, Glymour MA. Socioeconomic outcomes of women who receive and women who are denied wanted abortions. *Am J Public Health*. 2018;108(3): 407–413. https://doi.org/10.2105/AJPH.2017.304247r
3. De La Rue L. Intersectionality and resilience: updating how we address adolescent dating violence. *Am J Public Health*. 2019;109(10):1324–1325. https://doi.org/10.2105/AJPH.2019.305302

Caring for Military-Affiliated Transgender and Gender-Diverse Youths: A Call for Protections

David A. Klein, MD, MPH, Natasha A. Schvey, PhD, Thomas A. Baxter, DO, Noelle S. Larson, MD, and Christina M. Roberts, MD, MPH

ABOUT THE AUTHORS

David A. Klein is with the Departments of Family Medicine and Pediatrics, Uniformed Services University, Bethesda, MD, and the Department of Family Medicine, David Grant Medical Center, Travis Air Force Base, CA. Natasha A. Schvey is with the Department of Medical and Clinical Psychology, Uniformed Services University. Thomas A. Baxter is with the Department of Family Medicine, David Grant Medical Center, Travis Air Force Base, CA. Noelle S. Larson is with the Department of Pediatrics, Uniformed Services University, and the Department of Pediatrics, Walter Reed National Military Medical Center, Bethesda. Christina M. Roberts is with the Division of Adolescent Medicine, Children's Mercy Kansas City, and the Department of Pediatrics, University of Missouri-Kansas City School of Medicine.

Note. The opinions and assertions expressed herein are those of the authors and are not to be construed as reflecting the views of Uniformed Services University (USU), the Department of the Air Force, the Department of the Army, the US Department of Defense, or the US Government.

In the United States, 1.4% of youths between the ages of 13 and 17 years (or approximately 300 000 adolescents) identify as transgender or gender-diverse (TGD),[1] indicating that their gender identity, expression, or perception does not conform to the traditional gender roles and stereotypes associated with their assigned sex.[2] The recent increase in adolescents and young adults reporting a TGD identity is thought to be due to increased awareness of the full range of gender identities, social acceptance, and improvements in medical care.[1–4] Greater acceptance supports wellness.[2] Indeed, in a study examining the health of those referred to care between 2000 and 2016, those recently referred seemed to have better psychological functioning than those referred previously, whereas a similar proportion across the study time period chose to initiate gonadotropin-releasing hormone agonists (GnRH-a; used for puberty suppression) or gender-affirming hormones.[4]

Similar trends have occurred in the Military Health System (MHS). The number of new pediatric-age patients presenting for gender-affirming care in the MHS increased from 109 individuals a year in 2010 to over 600 a year in 2016.[3] In 2017, when gender-affirming medical care was included in the list of TRICARE benefits for about one year, at least 2500 children actively sought care for gender dysphoria through TRICARE Prime insurance at military or civilian treatment facilities, and 900 received GnRH-a or gender-affirming hormones.[3]

MILITARY-AFFILIATED YOUTHS

Approximately 918 000 youths aged 6 to 18 years have parents on active duty or ready reserve status, and one third of all military service members have children younger than 18 years.[5] Military-affiliated youths are faced with unique challenges and stressors, such as family separation and lack of parental support during training and deployments, heightened risk of anticipated or actual parental injury and death, and frequent geographic relocations, leading to disruptions of peer networks, scholastic environments, and health care.[6] The following sections examine the intersection between military-affiliated youths and gender-affirming care.

AFFIRMING MEDICAL CARE

Military dependent and nondependent TGD youths are at high risk for chronic stressors that may lead to poor mental health outcomes and risk-taking behaviors.[2,7] Compared with their siblings without gender dysphoria, TGD youths seen in the MHS had over five times greater odds of a mental health diagnosis and seven times greater odds of suicidal ideation or self-harm.[7] The stressors encountered by TGD youths include experiences of discrimination, harassment, stigma, and marginalization at multiple social-ecological levels, and unaddressed gender dysphoria.[2,8,9] Gender-affirming health care, such as puberty suppression and affirming hormones, mitigates these risks and optimizes patient-oriented outcomes, but many TGD youths have difficulty accessing services.[2,8–11]

AJPH March 2023, Vol 113, No. 3

BARRIERS TO CARE

Health care system barriers to gender-affirming treatment include discrimination, poor access, fear of mistreatment, and lack of trained clinicians willing to provide gender-affirming care.[9] Among military-affiliated physicians in the MHS, 87% indicated they did not have sufficient training to prescribe gender-affirming hormones to transgender adults and 53% said they would not prescribe gender-affirming hormones regardless of training.[12]

TGD youths in some states also face new legal barriers to accessing gender-affirming treatments.[13,14] Three states in the United States have outlawed all gender-affirming medical care for minors,[15] and one state government has classified it as child abuse. Sixteen state public insurance programs (e.g., Medicaid) that serve persons of low income and a disproportionate number of racial/ethnic minorities do not pay for gender-affirming care. Nineteen state legislatures are considering laws to ban aspects of gender-affirming medical care, including creating criminal penalties for parents and clinicians who seek out or provide gender-affirming care for minors.[14,15]

CRISIS IN GENDER-AFFIRMING CARE FOR MINORS

Legislative efforts to restrict gender-affirming care for youths have been described as a public health crisis. New state laws directly harm TGD adolescents by denying access to potentially life-saving medical care and further exacerbating health care inequities, health risk behaviors, and preventable deaths.[13,14]

These current legislative efforts, along with efforts to exclude gender identity from legal discrimination protections, restrict sports participation, and regulate bathroom use, also harm TGD youths indirectly by increasing exposure to discrimination, stigma, and marginalization that underlie the mental health disparities associated with gender dysphoria.[13,14] In a recent survey of 16 000 TGD civilian and military-affiliated youths aged 13 to 24 years across the United States, approximately half reported suicidality and 93% reported worry about transgender people being legally denied access to gender-affirming medical care.[8] In a recent study of parents of TGD youths, the majority feared that laws prohibiting care would worsen their child's mental health and decrease autonomy over medical decision-making for their children, including when they experience suicidality.[16]

These laws and regulations are especially harmful to youths who identify as Black, Indigenous, or people of color and those from disadvantaged backgrounds.[9] Such youths may be more likely to depend on state-financed medical coverage, which specifically excludes coverage for gender-affirming care, and many families may not have the resources to travel or relocate to access appropriate care.

LEGISLATION AND MILITARY-AFFILIATED YOUTHS

These restrictive state laws uniquely affect military TGD youths. Thirteen percent of the active-duty force lives in Texas, Arizona, Alabama, or Arkansas, states with the most restrictive laws on TGD-related care, and four of the five largest US military bases are located in states that have passed or are considering a ban on TGD-related care for minors.[5,15] Military-affiliated TGD youths with parents assigned to these states may have limited or no access to gender-affirming care. This will make it difficult for youths in the MHS to initiate or continue GnRH-a or gender-affirming hormones. Military families have limited autonomy in geographic assignment and may not have any choice about moving into states that deny their children this potentially life-saving care, or the resources and commander support to regularly travel out of state to obtain care.[5,15] Unwanted discontinuation of GnRH-a or gender-affirming hormones will lead to demonstrably harmful and nonsensical partial masculinization or feminization and may lead to depression, suicidality, poor quality of life, and other untoward outcomes.[17]

Providing gender-affirming care on a military base may not be a viable solution, as this may not protect parents or clinicians from criminal prosecution in states where rendering evidence-based, potentially lifesaving care to TGD youths is illegal or classified as child abuse. Similar to the case with local, non-military-affiliated clinicians, military clinicians who are qualified and willing to provide this care will be placed in a precarious and daunting situation when state laws conflict with ethical medical practice and the standard of care.[12,14,18] Clinicians, many of whom are concurrently serving honorably as active-duty officers in the United States Military, may be forced to choose between withholding recommended and medically necessary treatments to act in accordance with state law, and providing ethical and evidence-based treatment while facing legal or financial persecution, dishonorable military service, or allegations of child abuse. Families serving the country may face similar dilemmas and consequences.

State laws banning gender-affirming care for TGD youths are currently blocked by court injunctions as they progress through litigation. However, given the "Originalist" judicial philosophy of the majority of the current Supreme Court and the recent rejection of substantive due process protections for private health care decisions, it is plausible that these laws may soon be enforced.

THREATS TO MILITARY READINESS

The family unit is the foundation of a strong military force.[6] Threats to military-affiliated youths, parents, guardians, and clinicians are threats to military readiness. Service members frequently base their decision to reenlist or to extend military service on family factors, such as appropriate health care for dependents. Lack of health care services could affect the service member's retainability, morale, performance, operational readiness, recruitment, and overall health; optimal care can reduce stress.[6] For example, missed time at work, inability to deploy, and early return from deployment affect both home station and deployed missions.

ADDRESSING CONCERNS WITH GENDER-AFFIRMING CARE

In April 2022, a team of scholars at Yale University deconstructed the major arguments in which these laws are rooted.[19] State legislation overstates uncertainties in the medical literature supporting gender-affirming care, exaggerates associated risks, falsely claims that medical standards authorize sterilization for minors, and fails to consider and acknowledge the substantial benefits of gender-affirming treatment.[19] Current treatment guidelines describe the most effective and evidence-based treatment options, including the risks and benefits, based on four decades of research and clinical experience with TGD adolescents specifically, and substantially longer with TGD adults.[2,11]

These laws also assume that TGD adolescents and their parents are incapable of understanding the risks and benefits of gender-affirming medical care and then deciding what is in the youth's best interest. Prior research has found that children can begin participating in their medical decision-making as early as age seven years with gradual increases in decision-making capacity, and adolescents prefer shared decision-making.[2,20–22] Furthermore, military-affiliated adolescents who initiate gender-affirming hormones continue their medication at rates similar to or higher than those of adults, reflecting a similar understanding and tolerance of the effects of hormonal therapy.[23] Deontological and consequentialist reasoning, rooted in empirical evidence and human rights, suggests that youths with decisional capacity, in an informed consent model of care, have an inherent ability and right to consent to gender-affirming therapy.[20]

RECOMMENDATIONS: A PATH FORWARD

The United States Military has a long history of overcoming discriminatory policies affecting minoritized groups. In the case of gender diverse youths, the Department of Defense (DoD) can leverage its robust, intact systems to overcome evolving barriers to the provision of and access to care.

1. Publicly declare a position. The DoD through the Defense Health Agency (DHA) should publicly declare a gender-affirmative position on this issue, in accordance with the recommendations from multiple major medical societies that voice support for patients, parents, caregivers, and clinicians. Alternatively, a less public approach could involve a statement voicing support for insurance beneficiaries receiving evidence-based medical care informed by relevant medical organizations, while simultaneously fostering access to the full range of services. This may lead to less resistance and politicization, which could work against the overarching goals. However, affirming care has only recently become politicized; protection of gender-affirming medical care for military-affiliated TGD youths may require a declarative position without tolerance for personal biases, as the DoD has historically achieved for other minoritized groups.
2. Clarify boundaries. Clinicians who care for military-affiliated TGD youths should be familiar with relevant state laws that may limit provision of care, and available local and nonlocal resources. This information may fluctuate. To protect patients, parents, caregivers, and clinicians, current guidance should be updated regularly on relevant DHA Web sites for transparency. Nuanced information related to legalities by location of care (e.g., military treatment facilities, perhaps based on receipt of federal funding) and care provision rules (e.g., permissibility of telehealth or medical temporary duty based on physical location of patient or clinician) should be clearly

elucidated by DHA legal advisors. The DHA should also make a commitment to defending clinicians and families who render gender-affirming care to minors in accordance with DHA legal guidance from prosecution under state laws or policies that criminalize this care.

3. Leverage the Exceptional Family Member Program (EFMP). The DoD can codify specific and definitive policies through the EFMP, ensuring protections for youths with TGD identities, their families, and their health care teams. The United States Air Force has publicly discussed this strategy using command-driven personnel actions to move affected families to locations with available care; it has also discussed the robust use of the EFMP to prevent relocation of enrolled families to areas unable to provide indicated care because of state law.[24] The DoD must ensure that members of all military services have equitable benefits.
4. Use medical temporary duty judiciously. In states that permit travel for care across state lines, patients should be allowed access to medical temporary duty central funding to travel to states with a full range of care for specialized services. This model has been proven; military-affiliated patients from countries with barriers to gender-affirming services have temporarily visited a specialized military clinic in the United States periodically for care.[25] For example, an implantable puberty blocker, which is generally effective for at least two years, can be administered at a tertiary care military hospital, requiring only routine services easily accomplished in primary care over time. This could be a temporizing measure prior to relocation.
5. Foster telehealth capabilities. Telehealth has greatly evolved during the COVID-19 pandemic and has the potential to meaningfully increase access to care. The United States Air Force has piloted a telehealth program for transgender active-duty members and found high rates of patient satisfaction, suggesting the infrastructure is in place. Use of this platform will depend on details of specific state law, credentialing, and licensure.
6. Provide education and training. The extent to which gender-affirming care exists at each location of care varies.[12] The DHA, in partnership with the Uniformed Services University, can boost educational efforts for medical students, residents, and clinicians at military treatment facilities. Use of evidence-based clinical guidelines,[11] consultation with experts in military settings,[25] or civilian training programs (e.g., https://www.lgbtqiahealtheducation.org; https://www.wpath.org) can ensure relevant content.

Some well-intentioned military-affiliated clinicians may not be aware that a "watchful waiting" approach has a different risk profile than a gender-affirmative approach (which allows for gender identity exploration), and that "conversion therapy" is unethical, harmful, and generally illegal.[2] Patients may face "gatekeeping" and major delays in care, including protracted and pathologizing psychiatric evaluations that question patient motives. With proper training, clinicians can provide care in an informed-consent, longitudinal primary care model that integrates mental health, or multidisciplinary care, based on patient complexity and need, clinician comfort and training, state laws, and family preferences.[2,11]

7. Optimize treatment platforms. Clinicians serving military-affiliated TGD youths can ensure that their treatment platforms—such as their clinic environments, staff, and care recommendations—are welcoming, accessible, and evidence-based.[2] Facility commanders can be empowered to ensure institutional cultural responsiveness and humility among its clinical and support staff.
8. Sponsor research. Longitudinal research is needed to better understand long-term patient, family, and military outcomes associated with access to timely gender-affirming care. An investment in further educational and population-based health services research through military and civilian funding sources is warranted.

Military-affiliated youths with financial resources and strong parental support, as seen in other circumstances, may navigate the system to find appropriate solutions for lack of local care. Unfortunately, not all military-affiliated families or youths will have similar agency, leading to additional health care inequities among those without financial means or those at highest risk because of their multiple marginalization experiences. Low- or no-cost care through the TRICARE insurance program, including allowances for timely provision of GnRH-a—which can be cost-prohibitive for some nonaffiliated peers—already attenuates barriers to care. Additional supports from the DHA and local military commanders in the form of medical temporary duty sponsorship, as allowed, can further reduce risk.

A considerable worry is that for some youths with TGD identities, the stress of state laws and potential denial of necessary care will be insurmountable, resulting in poor mental health outcomes or suicide. The loss of these youths and the consequential suffering of the affected military families would be unfathomable and unacceptable. Those in immediate need can be referred to crisis resources (e.g., The Trevor Project; https://www.thetrevorproject.org); military-specific resources are available as well (https://modernmilitary.org/portfolio-items/milpride). In 2016, TRICARE formally approved coverage of care to TGD youths.[3] We believe the DoD can continue to lead in this domain. AJPH

CORRESPONDENCE

Correspondence should be sent to David A. Klein, MD, MPH, Department of Family Medicine, Uniformed Services University, 4301 Jones Bridge Rd, Bethesda, MD 20814 (e-mail: david.a.klein26.mil@health.mil). Reprints can be ordered at http://www.ajph.org by clicking the "Reprints" link.

PUBLICATION INFORMATION

Full Citation: Klein DA, Schvey NA, Baxter TA, Larson NS, Roberts CM. Caring for military-affiliated transgender and gender-diverse youths: a call for protections. *Am J Public Health*. 2023;113(3): 251–255.

Acceptance Date: October 20, 2022.

DOI: https://doi.org/10.2105/AJPH.2022.307163

CONTRIBUTORS

All authors sufficiently contributed to the conceptualization, design, drafting, and revision of content of this opinion editorial, and approved the final version.

ACKNOWLEDGMENTS

Children's Mercy Kansas City funded open access fees.

CONFLICTS OF INTEREST

The authors have no potential or actual conflicts of interest from funding or affiliation-related activities.

REFERENCES

1. Herman JL, Flores AR, O'Neill KK. How many adults identify as transgender in the United States? The Williams Institute. University of California, Los Angeles School of Law. 2022. Available at: https://williamsinstitute.law.ucla.edu/publications/trans-adults-united-states. Accessed November 7, 2022.
2. Rafferty J, Committee on Psychosocial Aspects of Child and Family Health, Committee on Adolescence, Section on Lesbian, Gay, Bisexual, and Transgender Health and Wellness, Yogman M, Baum R, et al. Ensuring comprehensive care and support for transgender and gender-diverse children and adolescents. *Pediatrics.* 2018;142(4): e20182162. https://doi.org/10.1542/peds.2018-2162
3. Klein DA, Roberts TA, Adirim TA, et al. Transgender children and adolescents receiving care in the US Military Health Care System. *JAMA Pediatr.* 2019;173(5):491–492. https://doi.org/10.1001/jamapediatrics.2019.0105
4. Arnoldussen M, Steensma TD, Popma A, van der Miesen AIR, Twisk JWR, de Vries ALC. Re-evaluation of the Dutch approach: are recently referred transgender youth different compared to earlier referrals? [erratum in *Eur Child Adolesc Psychiatry.* 2020;31(5):843.] *Eur Child Adolesc Psychiatry.* 2020; 29(6):803–811. https://doi.org/10.1007/s00787-019-01394-6
5. Dept of Defense, Office of the Deputy Assistant Secretary of Defense for Military Community and Family Policy. 2020 Demographics profile of the military community. 2021. Available at: https://www.militaryonesource.mil/data-research-and-statistics/military-community-demographics/2020-demographics-profile. Accessed November 7, 2022.
6. National Academies of Sciences, Engineering, and Medicine. *Strengthening the Military Family Readiness System for a Changing American Society.* Washington, DC: National Academies Press; 2019.
7. Hisle-Gorman E, Schvey NA, Adirim TA, et al. Mental healthcare utilization of transgender youth before and after affirming treatment. *J Sex Med.* 2021;18(8):1444–1454. https://doi.org/10.1016/j.jsxm.2021.05.014
8. The Trevor Project. National Survey on LGBTQ Youth. 2022. Available at: https://www.thetrevorproject.org/survey-2022/assets/static/trevor01_2022survey_final.pdf. Accessed November 7, 2022.
9. Chong LSH, Kerklaan J, Clarke S, et al. Experiences and perspectives of transgender youths in accessing health care: a systematic review. *JAMA Pediatr.* 2021;175(11):1159–1173. https://doi.org/10.1001/jamapediatrics.2021.2061
10. Chew D, Anderson J, Williams K, May T, Pang K. Hormonal treatment in young people with gender dysphoria: a systematic review. *Pediatrics.* 2018;141(4):e20173742. https://doi.org/10.1542/peds.2017-3742
11. Hembree WC, Cohen-Kettenis PT, Gooren L, et al. Endocrine treatment of gender-dysphoric/gender-incongruent persons: an Endocrine Society clinical practice guideline. *J Clin Endocrinol Metab.* 2017;102(11):3869–3903. https://doi.org/10.1210/jc.2017-01658
12. Schvey NA, Blubaugh I, Morettini A, Klein DA. Military family physicians' readiness for treating patients with gender dysphoria. *JAMA Intern Med.* 2017;177(5):727–729. https://doi.org/10.1001/jamainternmed.2017.0136
13. Barbee H, Deal C, Gonzales G. Anti-transgender legislation—a public health concern for transgender youth. *JAMA Pediatr.* 2022;176(2):125–126. https://doi.org/10.1001/jamapediatrics.2021.4483
14. Park BC, Das RK, Drolet BC. Increasing criminalization of gender-affirming care for transgender youths—a politically motivated crisis. *JAMA Pediatr.* 2021;175(12):1205–1206. https://doi.org/10.1001/jamapediatrics.2021.2969
15. Movement Advancement Project. Equality maps: healthcare laws and policies. 2022. Available at: https://www.lgbtmap.org/equality-maps/healthcare_laws_and_policies. Accessed November 7, 2022.
16. Kidd KM, Sequeira GM, Paglisotti T, et al. "This could mean death for my child": parent perspectives on laws banning gender-affirming care for transgender adolescents. *J Adolesc Health.* 2021; 68(6):1082–1088. https://doi.org/10.1016/j.jadohealth.2020.09.010
17. Wu SS, Raymer CA, Kaufman BR, Isakov R, Ferrando CA. The effect of preoperative gender affirming hormone therapy use on perioperative adverse events in transmasculine individuals undergoing masculinizing chest surgery for gender affirmation. *Aesthet Surg J.* 2022. https://doi.org/10.1093/asj/sjac091
18. Warling A, Keuroghlian AS. Clinician-level implications of bans on gender-affirming medical care for youth in the US. *JAMA Pediatr.* 2022;176(10): 963. https://doi.org/10.1001/jamapediatrics.2022.2771
19. Boulware SD, Kamody R, Luper L, et al. Biased science: the Texas and Alabama measures criminalizing medical treatment for transgender children and adolescents rely on inaccurate and misleading scientific claims. Yale University. 2022. Available at: https://medicine.yale.edu/lgbtqi/research/gender-affirming-care/biased-science. Accessed November 7, 2022.
20. Clark BA, Virani A. "This wasn't a split-second decision": an empirical ethical analysis of transgender youth capacity, rights, and authority to consent to hormone therapy. *J Bioeth Inq.* 2021; 18(1):151–164. https://doi.org/10.1007/s11673-020-10086-9
21. Dubin S, Lane M, Morrison S, et al. Medically assisted gender affirmation: when children and parents disagree. *J Med Ethics.* 2020;46(5):295–299. https://doi.org/10.1136/medethics-2019-105567
22. Vrouenraets LJJJ, de Vries ALC, de Vries MC, van der Miesen AIR, Hein IM. Assessing medical decision-making competence in transgender youth. *Pediatrics.* 2021;148(6):e2020049643. https://doi.org/10.1542/peds.2020-049643
23. Roberts CM, Klein DA, Adirim TA, Schvey NA, Hisle-Gorman E. Continuation of gender-affirming hormones among transgender adolescents and adults. *J Clin Endocrinol Metab.* 2022;107(9): e3937–e3943. https://doi.org/10.1210/clinem/dgac251
24. Youn S. Air Force offers help to LGBTQ personnel, families hurt by state laws. *Washington Post.* April 16, 2022. Available at: https://www.washingtonpost.com/politics/2022/04/16/air-force-lgbtq-laws-help-families. Accessed November 7, 2022.
25. Van Donge N, Schvey NA, Roberts TA, Klein DA. Transgender dependent adolescents in the US military health care system: demographics, treatments sought, and health care service utilization. *Mil Med.* 2019;184(5-6):e447–e454. https://doi.org/10.1093/milmed/usy264

The Future of Pharmacist-Delivered Status-Neutral HIV Prevention and Care

Paul J. Weidle, PharmD, MPH, John T. Brooks, MD, Sheila Salvant Valentine, JD, and Demetre Daskalakis, MD, MPH

ABOUT THE AUTHORS

Paul J. Weidle, John T. Brooks, Sheila Salvant-Valentine, and Demetre Daskalakis are with the Division of HIV Prevention, National Center for HIV, Viral Hepatitis, STD & TB Prevention, Centers for Disease Control and Prevention (CDC), Atlanta, GA.

Note. The findings and conclusions in this report are those of the authors and do not necessarily represent the official position of the CDC.

During 2019 in the United States, there were an estimated 1.2 million people with HIV and 34 800 new HIV infections, among which people belonging to minority ethnic and racial groups were disproportionally affected: 41% of new HIV diagnoses were among Black/African American people and 29% were among Hispanic/Latino people.[1] In February 2019, the US Department of Health and Human Services launched Ending the HIV Epidemic in the US, a multiagency initiative with four key strategies (Diagnose, Treat, Prevent, and Respond), which when implemented together can end the HIV epidemic in the United States by 2030.[2] Pharmacists and community pharmacies are and will continue to be an essential part of the public health and medical infrastructure needed to end the HIV epidemic. Pharmacists are positioned to facilitate linkage to mainstream health care by reaching people from racial and ethnic groups that are disproportionately affected by HIV. Durable pharmacist impact hinges on addressing policy and practice barriers to enable expanded pharmacy-based HIV services.[3] We call on leaders in public health, state and local health departments, professional organizations dedicated to addressing the needs of people with HIV, and community-based organizations to increase engagement with pharmacists and pharmacy associations within their jurisdiction. This could be accomplished, in part, by including them on HIV planning boards and utilizing their skills and availability to support a status-neutral approach to HIV services. These actions will not only help end the HIV epidemic in the United States, but will also help address the syndemic of HIV, viral hepatitis, sexually transmitted infections, and substance use disorder.

The value of pharmacists in public health response is exemplified by the transformational role they have undertaken during the COVID-19 pandemic,[4] delivering more than 250 million doses of COVID-19 immunizations by June 2022.[5] The foundation to respond had been laid by the pharmacy profession years earlier by strategically establishing pharmacies as venues for immunization services, in particular annual influenza vaccination.[6] Pharmacies can also be accessible sites to test and treat a variety of infectious diseases (e.g., influenza, COVID-19, group A streptococcus) under collaborative practice agreements with physicians or by using standing orders.[7] With these expanded capacities, pharmacists have addressed key components of public health, described more than 100 years ago by C. E. A. Winslow, as "the control of community infections" and "the organization of medical and nursing service for the early diagnosis and preventive treatment of disease."[8(p.30)] These components also address elements in the framework called for in the 2006 Policy Statement from the American Public Health Association on the role of the pharmacist in public health.[9] Much of what pharmacists do in the community and outpatient setting is clinical prevention provided to individuals through interventions that promote health and prevent disease—essential components of health care and public health.

Adoption of a status-neutral approach to HIV services—in which HIV testing serves as an entry point to services for people with either a positive or negative result—can improve prevention and care outcomes.[10] As front-line providers, pharmacists are well positioned to provide status-neutral care and advance the capacity to control HIV in the United States. People who receive a negative HIV test result can be offered powerful tools that prevent HIV, including preexposure prophylaxis and information about access to condoms, sexual health, and harm reduction services. People who receive a positive HIV test result can be quickly engaged in HIV primary care and prescribed effective treatment to help them rapidly achieve and durably maintain an undetectable viral load, which not only enables people with HIV to live long, healthy lives but prevents sexual HIV transmission.

Pharmacies are widely accessible, nonstigmatizing retail venues that could be more strategically leveraged to support a greater range of HIV prevention, care, and treatment services.[11] HIV self-testing has been passively supported through pharmacy-based sales of HIV self-test kits since they were first marketed in 2012. The advent of point-of-care tests for HIV and hepatitis C infection has created opportunities for pharmacists and community pharmacies to expand these prevention services more actively.[7] Health departments or community-based organizations could partner with pharmacies to increase distribution of HIV self-test kits or mail-in self-collection kits for HIV or for sexually transmitted infections through their extensive network in urban, suburban, and rural communities. Pharmacists have a well-established role supporting antiretroviral treatment of, and preexposure prophylaxis against, HIV infection through conventional practice of education and timely reminders for refilling prescriptions. Pharmacists' participation in HIV clinic-based settings, alongside other medical practitioners, has been supported by the Ryan White AIDS Care Program for decades.[12] Engaging community pharmacists as key players in a care team can increase retention in care and adherence to antiretroviral therapy and maintain viral suppression.[13] Pharmacists' involvement in preexposure prophylaxis care and delivery includes initiation of antivirals through standing orders or collaborative practice agreements with physicians, including through legislation in a growing number of states.[14] Pharmacists are critical for the timely dispensing of medications for postexposure prophylaxis against HIV infection in coordination with HIV prevention public health programs and clinicians.

Pharmacists have a major role in ensuring that HIV medications are effectively used. An emerging concept is to link medical claims data and pharmacy claims data for real-time public health action to identify people who have a diagnosis of HIV infection (medical claims) and ensure that they are filling prescriptions for antiretroviral therapy (pharmacy claims); the effectiveness of this approach is currently being determined.[15] Pharmacy claims data can also be used in real time to identify persons who have stopped or interrupted antiretroviral therapy and then, in turn, initiate a rapidly escalating series of interventions from the pharmacist, the medical provider, and the health department. In this way, public health can fulfill its function of ensuring that all people with HIV are taking antiretroviral therapy with resultant viral suppression. Using claims data in this manner requires logistical and administrative planning between different agencies and organizations, including the establishment of data use agreements. The pharmacist generates the data used for action and is integral to implementation of the intervention.

There are also underutilized opportunities for pharmacists to play a more prominent role in preventing the transmission of HIV and other infectious diseases through nonprescription syringe sales. More than 25% of persons who inject drugs obtain sterile syringes from pharmacies.[16] There are programs that provide a framework, developed by the state or local health department, that integrates syringe sales with HIV prevention counseling, and educates pharmacists and pharmacy staff on harm reduction strategies, syringe disposal, access to naloxone for opioid overdose treatment, and referrals for substance use disorder treatment.[17] Although most states allow for nonprescription syringe sales to people who inject drugs, implementation is typically left to the discretion of the pharmacist on duty. Without a clear strategy in place, conflict may arise between the public health need to prevent the spread of infectious diseases and personal beliefs regarding injection drug use, prior negative experiences, perceptions about persons with substance use disorder, and laws against distribution or possession of drug paraphernalia. Education and support for pharmacists, from both pharmacy management and policymakers, are needed for consistent application of nonprescription syringe sales in practice so pharmacists feel they are part of the solution to the prevention of infectious disease transmission, not part of the problem of the illicit drug use.

The Ending the HIV Epidemic in the US initiative provides a once-in-a-generation opportunity to control HIV in America. Doing so will require strengthening partnerships among public health leaders at the federal, state, and local levels, professional medical societies, HIV advocacy organizations, community-based organizations, health care providers, academic institutions, the business community, and other partners. Public health leaders, policymakers, pharmacists, and pharmacy associations should look for opportunities in their locality to expand the role of pharmacists in ending the HIV epidemic. AJPH

CORRESPONDENCE

Correspondence should be sent to Paul J. Weidle, PharmD, MPH, Centers for Disease Control and Prevention, 1600 Clifton Rd, MS USB-5, Atlanta GA, 30329 (e-mail: pweidle@cdc.gov). Reprints can be ordered at http://www.ajph.org by clicking the "Reprints" link.

PUBLICATION INFORMATION

Full Citation: Weidle PJ, Brooks JT, Valentine SS, Daskalakis D. The future of pharmacist-delivered status-neutral HIV prevention and care. *Am J Public Health*. 2023;113(3):256–258.

Acceptance Date: November 23, 2022.
DOI: https://doi.org/10.2105/AJPH.2022.307190

CONTRIBUTORS

All authors contributed to the writing and provided critical review of the editorial.

CONFLICTS OF INTEREST

The authors have no conflicts of interest to declare.

REFERENCES

1. Centers for Disease Control and Prevention. Estimated HIV incidence and prevalence in the United States, 2015–2019. HIV Surveillance Supplemental Report 2021;26(No. 1). May 2021. Available at: https://www.cdc.gov/hiv/pdf/library/reports/surveillance/cdc-hiv-surveillance-supplemental-report-vol-26-1.pdf. Accessed June 1, 2022.
2. Fauci AS, Redfield RR, Sigounas G, Weahkee M, Giroir BP. Ending the HIV epidemic: a plan for the United States. *JAMA*. 2019;321(9):844–845. https://doi.org/10.1001/jama.2019.1343
3. Crawford ND, Lewis CF, Moore R, Pietrandoni G, Weidle PJ. Examining the multilevel barriers to pharmacy-based HIV prevention and treatment services. *Sex Transm Dis*. 2022;49(11S suppl 2):S22–S25. https://doi.org/10.1097/OLQ.0000000000001643
4. Earl G, Cillessen L, Lyons-Burney H, et al. Pharmacists' role in infectious pandemics: illustration with COVID-19. In: Adejare A, Amin PD, Earl GL, eds. *Remington: The Science and Practice of Pharmacy*. 23rd ed. London, UK: Elsevier Inc; 2021:849–876. https://doi.org/10.1016/B978-0-12-820007-0.00064-7
5. Centers for Disease Control and Prevention. The federal retail pharmacy program for COVID-19 vaccination. Available at: https://www.cdc.gov/vaccines/covid-19/retail-pharmacy-program/index.html. Accessed June 6, 2022.
6. Centers for Disease Control and Prevention. Influenza vaccinations administered in pharmacies and physician medical offices, adults, United States. Available at: https://www.cdc.gov/flu/fluvaxview/dashboard/vaccination-administered.html. Accessed June 1, 2022.
7. Cillessen LM, Lyons-Burney H, Gubbins PO. Pharmacist use of point-of-care testing to improve access to care. In: Adejare A, Amin PD, Earl GL, eds. *Remington: The Science and Practice of Pharmacy*. 23rd ed. London, UK: Elsevier Inc; 2021:817–828. https://doi.org/10.1016/B978-0-12-820007-0.00046-5
8. Winslow CE. The untilled fields of public health. *Science*. 1920;51(1306):23–33. https://doi.org/10.1126/science.51.1306.23
9. American Public Health Association (APHA). The role of the pharmacist in public health. APHA policy no. 200614. 2006. Available at: //www.apha.org/policies-and-advocacy/public-health-policy-statements/policy-database/2014/07/07/13/05/the-role-of-the-pharmacist-in-public-health#:~:text=Prominent%20considerations%20of%20the%20role,patients%20and%20health%20team%20members. Accessed June 1, 2022.
10. The White House. National HIV/AIDS Strategy for the United States 2022–2025. 2021. Available at: https://www.hiv.gov/federal-response/national-hiv-aids-strategy/national-hiv-aids-strategy-2022-2025. Accessed June 1, 2022.
11. Myers JE, Farhat D, Guzman A, Arya V. Pharmacists in HIV prevention: an untapped potential. *Am J Public Health*. 2019;109(6):859–861. https://doi.org/10.2105/AJPH.2019.305057
12. Cantwell-McNelis K, James CW. Role of clinical pharmacists in outpatient HIV clinics. *Am J Health Syst Pharm*. 2002;59(5):447–452. https://doi.org/10.1093/ajhp/59.5.447
13. Byrd KK, Hou JG, Bush T, et al. Adherence and viral suppression among participants of the patient-centered Human Immunodeficiency Virus (HIV) Care Model Project: a collaboration between community-based pharmacists and HIV clinical providers. *Clin Infect Dis*. 2020;70(5):789–797. https://doi.org/10.1093/cid/ciz276
14. Farmer EK, Koren DE, Cha A, et al. The pharmacist's expanding role in HIV pre-exposure prophylaxis. *AIDS Patient Care STDS*. 2019;33(5):207–213. https://doi.org/10.1089/apc.2018.0294
15. Byrd KK, Camp NM, Iqbal K, Weidle PJ. Pharmacy data as an alternative data source for implementation of a data to care strategy. *J Acquir Immune Defic Syndr*. 2019;82(1):S53–S56. https://doi.org/10.1097/QAI.0000000000001969
16. Centers for Disease Control and Prevention. HIV infection risk, prevention, and testing behaviors among persons who inject drugs: National HIV Behavioral Surveillance, injection drug use, 23 US cities, 2018. HIV Surveillance Special Report 24. February 2020. Available at: https://www.cdc.gov/hiv/pdf/library/reports/surveillance/cdc-hiv-surveillance-special-report-number-24.pdf. Accessed June 1, 2022.
17. Anderson B, Mercier RC. The role of nonprescription syringe sales in ending the human immunodeficiency virus epidemic. *J Am Pharm Assoc (2003)*. 2022;62(4):1158–1161. https://doi.org/10.1016/j.japh.2022.02.017

Is the Goal of "The Healthiest Nation" Attainable or Desirable?

Namvar Zohoori, MD, PhD, MPH

ABOUT THE AUTHOR

Namvar Zohoori is professor of epidemiology at the Fay W. Boozman College of Public Health, University of Arkansas for Medical Sciences, and chief science officer at the Arkansas Department of Health, Little Rock.

Note. The views expressed are solely those of the author and do not necessarily reflect those of the Arkansas Department of Health.

For several years, the American Public Health Association (APHA) has had its sights set on the laudable and lofty goal of creating the healthiest nation in one generation. Since the announcement of the theme "Healthiest Nation 2030" for the 2015 National Public Health Week, this theme has been echoed in various forms and has served as a "clarion call to action" by APHA.[1] This focused attention to the nation's health has rightly generated many activities in several sectors in the nation and has identified and directed actions toward many important factors affecting health and health equity, such as racism, equal access to health care, and social determinants of health, among others.

At face value, the term "healthiest nation" may seem self-defining, but, in various publications, different definitions have been indirectly alluded to, such as making "the next United States generation the world's healthiest,"[1(p777)] or making the United States the "healthiest that we can be,"[2(pS219)] or stating that "the United States has the potential to become the healthiest nation in a healthier world."[3(p1)] Healthiest nation was also introduced as "an aspirational goal . . . that requires a culture change engaging all aspects of our society."[1(p777)] Therefore, variation in how healthiest nation is interpreted and understood is not trivial, because, to a large extent, the definitions set the goals, which, in turn, set the attitudes, strategies, and action steps toward achieving the goals. Moreover, the definition of healthiest nation also defines whether the goal is attainable, on the one hand, and desirable, on the other. In broad terms, healthiest nation can be defined in three ways, each of which should be examined in terms of its attainability and desirability.

THE HEALTHIEST IN THE WORLD

One definition for healthiest nation alluded to in various fora is "healthiest in the world."[1,3] Much has been written and said about the poor health ranking of the United States compared with other developed nations.[4–6] Given the many social, economic, and political factors that have contributed to this ranking for many decades, many of which continue to operate unabated, one can argue that this goal is unlikely to be attainable—that the United States can become the healthiest nation in the world by 2030, or even in one generation from now, as the goal has been variously promoted. However, regardless of whether this goal is attainable or not, we must also consider the implication and, thus, the desirability of such a goal. By definition, striving to become the healthiest nation in the world can indirectly promote the concepts of otherness and inequity. To strive to be the best in the world means striving to be better than others and leaving others behind—a goal that is not morally desirable or defensible. In any such race, there will only be one "winner" and many "losers," no matter how well everyone does.

Furthermore, striving to be the healthiest nation in the world is in many ways self-defeating. We have learned many lessons from the pandemic, but, if nothing else, we have learned that, especially when it comes to health in all its dimensions, no nation is an island. The pandemic has made it clear that nations and populations are more interdependent than ever for their health. Even before the pandemic, economic factors, trade, international travel, and migration made any nation's health dependent on health across the globe. The pandemic made that even clearer—as long as there are countries with substantial portions of their populations unvaccinated, there is fertile ground for new variants, or other infections, to emerge, putting all nations in peril. Therefore, no nation is safe or capable of winning the health race without all other nations having adequate levels of health—a goal that requires not a race as its core concept, but mutual international and intranational cooperation and collaboration.

Similarly, this definition can be self-defeating in another way—by creating a false sense of achievement and complacency. Being the healthiest among a group does not necessarily mean being healthy. An example from County Health Rankings may help illustrate this. An examination of states shows that in the state of Arkansas, for example, among its 75 counties, Benton County has consistently ranked at the top since 2010, scoring as the "healthiest" in the aggregate measures for both health outcomes and health factors, and as number 1 for both length and quality of life.[7] However, among 34 "peer" counties across the United States (as designated by County Health Rankings based on key demographic, social, and economic indicators), Benton County scores worse than 11 counties for premature deaths, 27 for poor or fair health, 26 for poor physical health, 22 for poor mental health, 6 for low birth weight, 22 for food environment, 20 for uninsured rate, 21 for children in poverty, 19 for reported violent crime rates, and 27 for air pollution, to name a few.[7] Being the healthiest among a group does not necessarily mean being healthy.

THE HEALTHIEST IT CAN BE

A second way in which heathiest nation can be interpreted is the "healthiest it can be."[2] This definition as a goal is desirable but arguably unattainable. Health is a continuum, with no currently definable or measurable endpoint, based on our current understanding. Becoming the healthiest nation we can be implies knowing the limits of health and, more importantly, how to get there. There are many dimensions to health, some of which are poorly studied or understood. We do not yet know or understand all the threats to health—natural or manmade. If we define health not only in physical terms but also in terms of mental, psychological, emotional, and spiritual factors, not only do we not know the limits of health, but we also certainly do not know how all these factors interact to produce ultimate health. Our understanding of such a state of health is changing continuously with new scientific developments. It is, therefore, not possible to be the healthiest we can be, because it is a currently undefinable ideal.

An alternative interpretation of this second definition might be the healthiest we can be "under the current circumstances." But that is a moving target, because that is, in fact, where we are at any given time—our current health status is the product of our current circumstances. These circumstances encompass our scientific knowledge, our social institutions and infrastructures, and our political will—that is, our current health status is the result of a combination of not only what we know but also how we have chosen, or been forced, to apply that knowledge to the operation of our overall health care and public health systems in all their facets. And the result of all that is the level of health we currently have. It is only by changing these current, mostly social and political, circumstances that we can become healthier than we are now.

THE HEALTHIEST IT HAS EVER BEEN

The term healthiest nation can be defined in yet a third way that is both attainable and desirable: the "healthiest it has ever been." This definition recognizes the fact that, no matter how healthy we have ever been as a nation, we can always be healthier. There is no limit to that. We can always go a step further, little by little, day by day. And that is potentially attainable.

This definition is also desirable. With this definition, our only "competition" is ourselves, and that means that every nation can be the healthiest nation and continue to strive for better. It puts every nation on its own desirable trajectory of continuous health improvement without having to leave other nations behind to achieve it. It also embodies the concept of continuous health maintenance and guarding against losing ground. Another benefit of this definition as a goal is that aid, assistance, and collaborations with other nations need not be at the expense of jeopardizing our own standing. We can all help each other on the path to health improvement and still maintain our own healthiest status, no matter how healthy other nations become as a result.

However, the desirability of this definition comes with a caveat. Even under this definition, the title of healthiest nation can hide significant levels of disparity within a nation. It is not enough for any nation to be able to say it is the healthiest it has ever been if all segments of the population within the nation cannot say the same thing. That is, it is not enough for average national health indicators to improve if that improvement is not experienced by all segments of society. This conceptualization requires us to think and plan differently about becoming the healthiest nation. Instead of trying to raise the national average—which statistically can be achieved by raising even higher the health of only those already doing the best, or raising their levels more than those at the lower end of the scale—it asks us to pay particular and focused attention to those at the bottom, and to raise their health levels at an even higher rate to close any gaps. In fact, it is likely that in many cases the national average can be raised even faster and more significantly by bringing up the lowest levels first and faster. This approach to the definition, then, requires us to not leave anyone behind, or increase the gap, in the quest to be the healthiest nation we have ever been.

CONCLUSIONS

Even with the attainable and desirable definition of the "healthiest we have ever been," we have, unfortunately, failed over the past few years. From 2019 to 2021, life expectancy at birth in the United States had its biggest two-year decline since 1921–1923, bringing us to 76.1 years, the lowest level since 1996.[8] The largest contributors to this decline were COVID-19; increases in deaths from accidents, suicides, and unintentional injuries, including drug overdose deaths; and chronic diseases, all of which have shown disparities along gender, racial, and ethnic lines. This does not bode well for attaining our healthiest nation goal, regardless of what definition we choose to use.

This setback notwithstanding, as a nation, we have made great strides. The public health community can be proud of important campaigns and programs that have led to major gains in health and life expectancy in the United States since the latter part of the 19th century. These campaigns have spanned several decades in the areas of infectious diseases, sanitation, water quality, vaccines and immunizations, tobacco prevention and cessation, trauma systems, and maternal and child health, among others. Initiatives like the decades-long Department of Health and Human Services' Healthy People campaign, and the more recent APHA's Healthiest Nation 2030—the focus of this editorial—have impelled us to go further as a nation. These campaigns, and many others, are now calling on us to pay more attention to health equity, and that requires us to think more deliberately and inclusively about how we conceptualize being healthy and how we strive to become the healthiest nation in a way that is both attainable and desirable. AJPH

CORRESPONDENCE

Correspondence should be sent to Namvar Zohoori, MD, PhD, MPH, Arkansas Department of Health, 4815 W Markham St, Slot 60, Little Rock, AR 72207 (e-mail: namvar.zohoori@arkansas.gov). Reprints can be ordered at https://ajph.org by clicking the "Reprints" link.

PUBLICATION INFORMATION

Full Citation: Zohoori N. Is the goal of "the healthiest nation" attainable or desirable? *Am J Public Health*. 2023;113(3):259–261.

Acceptance Date: December 10, 2022.

DOI: https://doi.org/10.2105/AJPH.2022.307204

ACKNOWLEDGMENTS

The author would like to thank Joseph Bates, MD, and Austin Porter III, DrPH, for their comments on an earlier draft.

CONFLICTS OF INTEREST

The author has no conflicts of interest to declare.

REFERENCES

1. Benjamin GC. Building a movement to be the healthiest nation. *Am J Public Health*. 2016; 106(5):777. https://doi.org/10.2105/AJPH.2016.303196
2. Benjamin GC. Becoming the healthiest nation: the role of Healthy People 2030. *J Public Health Manag Pract*. 2021;27(suppl 6):S218–S219. https://doi.org/10.1097/PHH.0000000000001417
3. Association of State and Territorial Health Officials. A transformed health system in the 21st century white paper. Available at: https://www.astho.org/globalassets/pdf/transformed-health-system-white-paper.pdf. Accessed September 20, 2022.
4. Tikkanen R, Abrams MK. US health care from a global perspective, 2019: higher spending, worse outcomes? Commonwealth Fund. January 30, 2020. Available at: https://www.commonwealthfund.org/publications/issue-briefs/2020/jan/us-health-care-global-perspective-2019. Accessed September 20, 2022.
5. Schneider EC, Shah A, Doty MM, et al. Mirror, mirror 2021: reflecting poorly. Health care in the US compared to other high-income countries. Commonwealth Fund. August 4, 2021. Available at: https://www.commonwealthfund.org/publications/fund-reports/2021/aug/mirror-mirror-2021-reflecting-poorly. Accessed September 20, 2022.
6. Kaiser Family Foundation. How does health spending in the US compare to other countries? January 21, 2022. Available at: https://www.kff.org/slideshow/health-spending-in-the-u-s-as-compared-to-other-countries-slideshow. Accessed September 20, 2022.
7. Muganda C, Hoffelder J, Olson-Williams H, et al. County Health Rankings state report 2022. University of Wisconsin. 2022. Available at: https://www.countyhealthrankings.org. Accessed September 20, 2022.
8. Centers for Disease Control and Prevention, National Center for Health Statistics. Life expectancy in the U.S. dropped for the second year in a row in 2021. August 31, 2022. Available at: https://www.cdc.gov/nchs/pressroom/nchs_press_releases/2022/20220831.htm. Accessed November 29, 2022.

Achieving Healthiest Nation Status Is Both Attainable and Desirable

Georges C. Benjamin, MD

ABOUT THE AUTHOR

Georges C. Benjamin is executive director of the American Public Health Association.

This issue of *AJPH* contains a thoughtful commentary by Zohoori (p. 259) about the issues surrounding the American Public Health Association (APHA) strategic vision to create the healthiest nation in one generation. Achieving healthiest nation status is indeed an ambitious, audacious goal. But those in public health have the responsibility of being the chief health strategists for the nation's health, and if we are to accept that responsibility, we must set a goal that meets the highest possible vision of that challenge. It is true that the United States spends much more on health care than do other high-income countries.[1] Despite this level of investment, we have poorer overall health system performance and poorer overall health outcomes.[2] History has shown that the United States has the capacity to be an exemplar in anything that it puts its national will, creativity, and enormous resources to.

When the APHA originally took as our strategic direction becoming the national leader in health improvement, we understood the enormous challenge it would be. We also understood that we as an association could not do it alone. We took seriously the 1988 Institute of Medicine report's description of the mission of public health as "fulfilling society's interest in assuring conditions in which people can be healthy" (https://www.ncbi.nlm.nih.gov/books/NBK218215). To that end, the APHA has worked on building the political will to make becoming the healthiest nation a goal and has advocated adequate resources for a robust and adequately resourced national public health system to achieve this goal. During National Public Health Week in April 2016, which focused on becoming the healthiest nation by 2030, we brought attention to this effort.[3] We have now built a movement through social media called Generation Public Health that has more than one million individuals dedicated to improving the public's health and that we believe is building the political will for change.

There have clearly been setbacks along the way. Epidemics of obesity, opioids, and now COVID-19 have stymied this effort, resulting in continued decreases in life expectancy over the past few years. For 2020, life expectancy fell an additional 0.6 year because of increases in mortality attributable to "COVID-19, unintentional injuries, chronic liver disease and cirrhosis, suicide, and homicide."[4(p6)] Nevertheless, the APHA continues to believe healthiest nation status is achievable. Whether it is international sports, scientific achievement, or the space race, Americans are a competitive people. We like to win. Imagine what we could achieve if our national will was focused on having healthy people in healthy communities. What if we received the best value for our enormous fiscal investment in health by ensuring universal health coverage, increasing our focus on prevention and primary care, and addressing with intention the social determinants of health? What if we truly strove to achieve equity in health status?

Following this pathway would lead us to success. We have work to do to reverse several years of declining life expectancy. Choosing to take the pathway toward becoming the healthiest nation is desirable and attainable and is, in fact, our only choice. AJPH

CORRESPONDENCE

Correspondence should be sent to Georges C. Benjamin, Executive Director, American Public Health Association, 800 I St, NW, Washington, DC 20001 (e-mail: georges.benjamin@apha.org). Reprints can be ordered at http://www.ajph.org by clicking the "Reprints" link.

PUBLICATION INFORMATION

Full Citation: Benjamin GC. Achieving healthiest nation status is both attainable and desirable. *Am J Public Health*. 2023;113(3):262.

Acceptance Date: January 4, 2023.

DOI: https://doi.org/10.2105/AJPH.2023.307219

CONFLICTS OF INTEREST

The author has no conflicts of interest to declare.

REFERENCES

1. Wager E, Ortaliza J, Cox C. How does health spending in the US compare to other countries? January 21, 2022. Available at: https://www.healthsystemtracker.org/chart-collection/health-spending-u-s-compare-countries-2. Accessed January 5, 2023.
2. Schneider EC, Shah A, Doty MM, Tikkanen R, Fields K, Williams RD II. Mirror, mirror 2021: reflecting poorly: health care in the U.S. compared to other high-income countries. August 4, 2021. Available at: https://www.commonwealthfund.org/publications/fund-reports/2021/aug/mirror-mirror-2021-reflecting-poorly. Accessed January 5, 2023.
3. Benjamin GC. Building a movement to be the healthiest nation. *Am J Public Health*. 2016;106(5):777. https://doi.org/10.2105/AJPH.2016.303196
4. Xu J, Murphy SL, Kochanek KD, Arias E. Mortality in the United States, 2021. *NCHS Data Brief*. 2022;(456):1–8.

A Community-Engaged Social Marketing Campaign to Promote Equitable Access to COVID-19 Services Among Latino Immigrants

Harita S. Shah, MD, Alejandra Flores Miller, Cui Yang, PhD, Suzanne M. Grieb, PhD, MSPH, Mitchell Lipke, Benjamin F. Bigelow, Katherine H. Phillips, MSN, MPH, Pedro Palomino, and Kathleen R. Page, MD

To address disparities in COVID-19 outcomes among Latinos with limited English proficiency in Maryland, our team developed a culturally congruent intervention that coupled a statewide social marketing campaign with community-based COVID-19 services. In the first year, we reached 305 122 people through social media advertisements and had 9607 visitors to the Web site. Social marketing campaigns represent an opportunity to promote COVID-19 testing and vaccine uptake among Latino populations, especially when they are paired with community services that simultaneously address structural barriers to care. (*Am J Public Health*. 2023;113(3):263–266. https://doi.org/10.2105/AJPH.2022.307191)

AJPH March 2023, Vol 113, No. 3

The COVID-19 pandemic has disproportionately affected Latino populations in the United States, with Latinos accounting for 18% of the US population but 27% of all COVID-19 cases in 2020.[1] A number of factors (e.g., occupational exposures, higher household occupancy, lack of insurance, limited English proficiency) have led to Latino immigrant communities experiencing a disproportionate burden of COVID-19 infections and mortality.[2,3] Social marketing interventions have been shown to be effective in reaching populations with barriers to accessing traditional health care settings, including Latino populations.[4,5] We sought to address disparities in COVID-19 testing and vaccination by coupling a social marketing campaign with accessible community-based COVID-19 services in Maryland.

INTERVENTION AND IMPLEMENTATION

Our team developed the *Mejor Vive Sin Duda* (Better to Live Without Doubt) social marketing intervention (hereafter referred to as *Sin Duda*) through community-based participatory research.[6] The *Sin Duda* campaign was coupled with community health worker (CHW) navigation and community-based COVID-19 services to simultaneously address structural barriers to care. The campaign evolved with the COVID-19 pandemic in three main iterations focused on COVID-19 testing, COVID-19 vaccination, and COVID-19 home tests and treatment.

Our team began by developing accessible COVID-19 testing and vaccination services in partnership with local community-based organizations (CBOs).[7,8] Services included free community-based events conducted twice a week as well as a COVID-19 hotline for Latinos, each staffed by a team of bilingual CHWs. We then developed and implemented the *Sin Duda* campaign, guided by a community advisory board at each stage. The campaign name was developed through a crowdsourcing open contest to incorporate community input.[9]

The campaign's "call to action" was to visit the project Web site (www.sinduda.org), which included COVID-19 information in English and Spanish and options to request CHW navigation to COVID-19 services via a Qualtrics form or the hotline. The campaign content was designed to have not only linguistic concordance but also cultural congruence, incorporating cultural beliefs from diverse countries of origin guided by input from Latino community members and team members (e.g., the community advisory board, CHWs, media designers).

Advertisements were distributed through Facebook and Instagram (Figure A, available as a supplement to the online version of this article at http://www.ajph.org) as well as Facebook and WhatsApp CBO groups. The campaign's testing and vaccination phases each consisted of two social media pushes six to eight weeks in duration that featured four to six new advertisements to capture users' attention and prevent advertisement fatigue. Finally, we included offline advertisements (e.g., radio, billboards) for two- to three-month periods to build campaign recognition and reach those without social media access.

PLACE, TIME, AND PERSONS

The *Sin Duda* campaign launched across Maryland on March 1, 2021, and remains active. Here we present the first year of data (through March 1, 2022), which included the COVID-19 testing and COVID-19 vaccination iterations. Services are designed to meet the needs of Latino adults and children in Maryland, with a focus on those with limited English proficiency.

PURPOSE

The *Sin Duda* campaign seeks to improve COVID-19 outcomes among Latino populations with barriers to accessing traditional health care settings by (1) promoting awareness and uptake of community-based COVID-19 services, (2) disseminating timely, evidence-based COVID-19 information to combat misinformation, and (3) empowering community members through community-based participatory research and partnerships with CBOs.

EVALUATION AND ADVERSE EFFECTS

Reach was evaluated via online metrics and surveys conducted at 30 different community-based venues (e.g., churches, consulates, parks) from March to July 2022. Participants were asked to provide information on demographic characteristics and were asked whether and how they had seen or heard of *Sin Duda*. We report descriptive statistics from the first year of the campaign and the survey period.

From March 1, 2021, to March 1, 2022, the *Sin Duda* campaign reached 305 122 people through paid advertisements on Facebook and Instagram (as measured by these platforms). Further organic (unpaid) reach was achieved via posts on CBO WhatsApp groups and social media pages. For context, the Latino adult population in Maryland is estimated at 492 262 residents; of these individuals, 274 298 are estimated to be foreign born.[10] Figure A displays examples of advertisements with high performance as defined by social media industry benchmarks (e.g., reach, click-through rates).

During the first year, we had 9607 unique visitors to the project Web site (Table 1). After the addition of a vaccination-focused page in May 2021, there were 1075 Web site requests for COVID-19 vaccinations. Requests via telephone calls were more common than requests via Qualtrics forms.

Among the 424 survey respondents, 29% (n = 121) indicated they had seen or heard of the *Sin Duda* campaign.

TABLE 1— Characteristics of *Mejor Vive Sin Duda* Web Site Users: Maryland, March 1, 2021–March 1, 2022

	No. (%)
Referral source	
Social media advertisement	7321 (76)
Direct URL entry	1830 (19)
Google or other Web site	456 (5)
Language	
Spanish	5283 (55)
English	4324 (45)
Method of access	
Mobile phone	7686 (80)
Desktop computer	1825 (19)
Tablet computer	96 (1)
Location	
Maryland	6965 (73)
Outside of Maryland	2642 (27)
Means of request for COVID-19 vaccine services[a]	
Call to Baltimore Esperanza Center hotline	408 (38)
Call to Maryland vaccine hotline	260 (24)
Qualtrics form	407 (38)

Note. The sample size was 9607.
[a]May 20, 2021, to March 1, 2022 (n = 1075).

Facebook was the most common means of exposure (n = 102; 84% of those exposed), followed by WhatsApp (n = 64; 53%). Of the respondents exposed to the campaign, 61% (n = 74) reported that it influenced their decision to get vaccinated, 32% (n = 39) reported that it helped them understand how to obtain vaccination or testing, 12% (n = 14) reported that it influenced their decision to undergo COVID-19 testing, and 16% (n = 19) reported that it did not influence them.

There were no known adverse effects stemming from this intervention.

SUSTAINABILITY

We adapted the *Sin Duda* campaign to focus on home-based testing and linkage to COVID-19 treatment. As a result of improved testing and vaccine availability via state and local agencies, CHW navigation has shifted to include these services. After the current funding period, the Web site will remain a resource to Maryland communities as long as it is relevant in terms of the COVID-19 pandemic.

PUBLIC HEALTH SIGNIFICANCE

The *Sin Duda* campaign is one of the first social marketing interventions to promote COVID-19 services in Latino communities that are home to residents with limited English proficiency. Community engagement at each project stage was key to ensuring relevant and effective content. In its first year, the campaign reached 305 122 Latino individuals across Maryland, and survey data demonstrated comparable reach to previous interventions.[5] The majority of survey respondents exposed to the campaign reported that it influenced their decision to get vaccinated or helped them understand how to obtain services. However, 71% of survey respondents did not report campaign exposure, highlighting the need for further efforts to more effectively reach underserved populations.

By coupling the reach of social marketing with community-based services to address systemic barriers to care, we were able to serve Latino populations in Maryland in multiple ways. First, the campaign increased awareness of local COVID-19 services, thereby expanding the potential client base for COVID-19 testing and vaccination. Second, social marketing provided a nimble medium to disseminate timely, evidence-based COVID-19 information. Third, *Sin Duda* provided culturally congruent avenues of communication for Latino individuals outside of traditional health care settings.

Our experience may inform future social marketing interventions seeking to reach underserved populations. Although Instagram and Tiktok have eclipsed platforms such as Facebook and WhatsApp among younger and English-speaking populations, CBO Facebook and WhatsApp groups have proven key in reaching Latino immigrant adults.[5,11] This represents an ongoing opportunity to financially support local CBOs while distributing information through trusted community channels.

In terms of content, the highest performing advertisements featured themes of self-efficacy and collective efficacy.[9] Media coverage of COVID-19 in Latino populations has often focused on vaccine hesitancy.[12] Our team has found that, in addition to addressing intersectional factors that contribute to vaccine hesitancy, strength-based messaging can be more effective than deficit-based messaging. Future social marketing interventions can tailor lessons learned from the *Sin Duda* campaign to local communities and should incorporate access to culturally congruent services to address systemic barriers to care. AJPH

ABOUT THE AUTHORS

Harita S. Shah is with the Department of Medicine, University of Chicago, Chicago, IL. Alejandra Flores Miller, Suzanne M. Grieb, Mitchell Lipke, Benjamin F. Bigelow, and Kathleen R. Page are with the Johns Hopkins University School of Medicine, Baltimore, MD. Cui Yang is with the Rutgers School of Public Health, Piscataway, NJ. Katherine H. Phillips is with the Esperanza Center, Baltimore, MD. Pedro Palomino is with Somos Baltimore Latino, Baltimore, MD.

CORRESPONDENCE

Correspondence should be sent to Harita S. Shah, MD, University of Chicago, 5841 S Maryland Ave, MC 3051, Chicago, IL 60637 (e-mail: harita.shah@bsd.uchicago.edu). Reprints can be ordered at http://www.ajph.org by clicking the "Reprints" link.

PUBLICATION INFORMATION

Full Citation: Shah HS, Miller AF, Yang C, et al. A community-engaged social marketing campaign to promote equitable access to COVID-19 services among Latino immigrants. *Am J Public Health*. 2023;113(3):263–266.

Acceptance Date: November 23, 2022.

DOI: https://doi.org/10.2105/AJPH.2022.307191

CONTRIBUTORS

H. S. Shah led the social marketing intervention development and implementation and the writing of the article. A. Flores Miller, C. Yang, S. M. Grieb, and K. R. Page served as project mentors and guided intervention development and implementation with the involvement of the community advisory board. M. Lipke provided survey data and analysis. B. F. Bigelow led the implementation of community-based services. K. H. Phillips and P. Palomino were key community-based implementation partners. All of the authors contributed to the study design, research process, and critical editing of the article.

ACKNOWLEDGMENTS

Research reported in this Rapid Acceleration of Diagnostics—Underserved Populations (RADx-UP) publication was supported by the National Institutes of Health (award R01DA045556-04S1).

We are grateful for the contributions of Altavista Studios, Ana Ortega Meza, Melissa Cuesta, the Esperanza Center, Somos Baltimore Latino, and the members of our community advisory board.

Note. The content is solely the responsibility of the authors and does not necessarily represent the official views of the National Institutes of Health.

CONFLICTS OF INTEREST

The authors have no potential or actual conflicts of interest to disclose.

HUMAN PARTICIPANT PROTECTION

This project was deemed exempt by the Johns Hopkins University School of Medicine institutional review board because it involved surveys with no more than minimal risk to participants.

REFERENCES

1. Centers for Disease Control and Prevention (CDC). Demographic trends of COVID-19 cases and deaths in the US reported to CDC: cases by race/ethnicity; deaths by race/ethnicity; cases by age group; deaths by age group; cases by sex; deaths by sex. Available at: https://stacks.cdc.gov/view/cdc/99332. Accessed March 29, 2022.
2. Poulson M, Neufeld M, Geary A, et al. Intersectional disparities among Hispanic groups in COVID-19 outcomes. *J Immigr Minor Health.* 2021;23(1):4–10. https://doi.org/10.1007/s10903-020-01111-5
3. Page KR, Flores-Miller A. Lessons we've learned—COVID-19 and the undocumented Latinx community. *N Engl J Med.* 2021;384(1):5–7. https://doi.org/10.1056/NEJMp2024897
4. Hunt IV, Dunn T, Mahoney M, Chen M, Nava V, Linos E. A social media–based public health campaign encouraging COVID-19 vaccination across the United States. *Am J Public Health.* 2022;112(9):1253–1256. https://doi.org/10.2105/AJPH.2022.306934
5. Shah HS, Dolwick Grieb SM, Flores-Miller A, Greenbaum A, Castellanos-Aguirre J, Page KR. *Sólo Se Vive Una Vez*: the implementation and reach of an HIV screening campaign for Latinx immigrants. *AIDS Educ Prev.* 2020;32(3):229–242. https://doi.org/10.1521/aeap.2020.32.3.229
6. Calva A, Matthew RA, Orpinas P. Overcoming barriers: practical strategies to assess Latinos living in low-income communities. *Health Promot Pract.* 2020;21(3):355–362. https://doi.org/10.1177/1524839919837975
7. Bigelow BF, Saxton RE, Flores-Miller A, et al. Community testing and SARS-CoV-2 rates for Latinxs in Baltimore. *Am J Prev Med.* 2021;60(6):e281–e286. https://doi.org/10.1016/j.amepre.2021.01.005
8. Bigelow BF, Saxton RE, Martínez DA, et al. High uptake and series completion of COVID-19 vaccine at community-based vaccination for Latinos with limited English proficiency. *J Public Health Manag Pract.* 2022;28(6):E789–E794. https://doi.org/10.1097/PHH.0000000000001625
9. Shah HS, Dolwick Grieb SM, Flores-Miller A, et al. A crowdsourcing open contest to design a Latino-specific COVID-19 campaign: a mixed methods analysis. *JMIR Form Res.* 2022;6(5):e35764. https://doi.org/10.2196/35764
10. US Census Bureau. Explore census data. Available at: https://data.census.gov. Accessed March 29, 2022.
11. Powell R, Rosenthal J, August EM, et al. Ante La Duda, Pregunta: a social marketing campaign to improve contraceptive access during a public health emergency. *Health Commun.* 2022;37(2):177–184. https://doi.org/10.1080/10410236.2020.1828534
12. Wan W. Coronavirus vaccines face trust gap in black and Latino communities, study finds. Available at: https://www.washingtonpost.com/health/2020/11/23/covid-vaccine-hesitancy. Accessed March 29, 2022.

The Challenges to Public Health Law in the Aftermath of COVID-19

Wendy E. Parmet, JD, and Paul C. Erwin, MD, DrPH

ABOUT THE AUTHORS

Wendy E. Parmet is with the Center for Health Policy & Law, Northeastern University, Boston, MA. Paul C. Erwin is with the School of Public Health, University of Alabama at Birmingham. Both authors are associate editors of AJPH.

See also Wiley, p. 269, Gostin, p. 272, Hodge et al., p. 275, Parmet and Khalik, p. 280, and Platt et al., p. 288.

Scholars have come to recognize that law operates as a social determinant of health.[1] That has been especially apparent since the start of the COVID-19 pandemic, during which federal and state laws abetted the rapid development and deployment of lifesaving vaccines, supported health care systems that faced unprecedented strain, and provided critical economic support to individuals and businesses. State and local laws also helped enforce physical distancing, required masking, and in some instances mandated vaccination. Taken together, these legal responses undoubtedly saved lives and prevented economic disaster.[2,3]

The pandemic, however, also highlighted the limit of law's capacity to support public health. As early as 2021, it was apparent that "for law to be effective, there must be strong leadership, ample resources fairly distributed, and the public's trust."[4(p.48)] Two years later, as the articles in this special section document, it is also evident that the use of law to protect the public's health faces considerable political and judicial resistance. As these articles show, this pushback raises serious questions about law's continued capacity to protect population health and address health inequities moving forward.

In their opinion editorial, Hodge et al. (p. 275) assess the state of public health emergency laws before, during, and after the pandemic. They begin by discussing the 2001 Model State Emergency Health Powers Act, which was designed to provide officials with a range of authorities they might need during a pandemic. After showing how the model act foresaw the types of measures that states used in response to COVID-19, they explain that most states relied on general emergency laws rather than their specific public health powers during the pandemic. Regardless, state orders faced resistance in both the political and judicial arenas, in part because of what the authors term COVID-19 "denialism." They conclude by highlighting several responses to that denialism and calling for efforts to reform public health laws to make them more robust and limit "denialist political influences."

Parmet and Khalik (p. 280) describe the challenges to public health and elected officials' use of emergency powers and other legal authorities in their analysis of the more than 1000 judicial decisions related to or precipitated by COVID-19 between March 1, 2020, and July 1, 2022. The decisions were broadly categorized by legal claims relating to (1) individual rights, (2) scope of authority, and (3) administrative procedures. Individual rights claims were the most common challenges, including claims alleging violations of the right to due process and equal protection under the Fourteenth Amendment (e.g., shuttering or restricting some but not all businesses), the Second Amendment (e.g., closing gun stores or shooting ranges), and the Free Exercise Clause of the First Amendment (e.g., limiting or banning in-person worship).

Many of the challenges to scope of authority pertained to measures that were not explicitly authorized by statute, including cases challenging governors' authority to declare or extend states of emergency and the eviction moratorium of the Centers for Disease Control and Prevention (CDC). Challenges to administrative procedures included claims that uses of emergency powers bypassed the usual rulemaking processes. Although smallest in number of the three categories of legal claims, courts were more likely to rule in favor of plaintiffs (33 of 85 relevant decisions) in challenges to administrative procedures than in the other two categories. The analysis of these judicial decisions indicates that, in contrast to earlier periods, public health officials can no longer assume that courts will give them the benefit of doubt when they impose measures to control or mitigate disease. This is especially evident in the Supreme Court's decisions regarding the free exercise of religion.

Platt et al. (p. 288) review 1531 bills addressing emergency health authority that were introduced by state legislators between January 1, 2021, and May 20, 2022. The authors group these bills

AJPH March 2023, Vol 113, No. 3

into six categories: limiting public health authority, expanding public health authority, shifting public health authority responsibility, limiting federal laws, regulating emergency measures, and preempting emergency measures. Of the 1531 bills introduced, 191 were passed by 43 states and the District of Columbia during the observation period, including 65 laws limiting public health authority (by limiting the authority of governors, other state officials, or local health officials), 17 expanding authority, 163 regulating the use of public health authority, and 30 preempting local use of public health measures. Although the authors found no significant difference in political party affiliation for bills that were introduced, there was a striking difference in affiliation for the outcomes of these bills: all states but one (Connecticut) that enacted one or more restrictive public health laws were controlled by Republican legislators.

The authors characterize the environment of this outpouring of legislative activity in clear language:

> Given the politicization of public health work during COVID-19, and the social shock of the pandemic, rapid and substantial changes to public health authority seem to reflect the frustration and irritation of a painful experience rather than a well-considered and evidence informed analysis of the authority health agencies need and what factors—leadership, funding, and other resources—drive strong health agency performance. (p. 294)

In her editorial, Wiley (p. 269) looks forward to the Supreme Court's 2022–2023 term. After noting that the cases the court will decide in 2023 are likely to have a "less direct and less dramatic" effect on health than the major decisions of 2022, Wiley discusses several pending cases that may have significant implications for health. Among them are cases regarding the ability of Medicaid beneficiaries and providers to enforce federal requirements for that program, the right of businesses to refuse to comply with civil rights laws when doing so conflicts with their self-expression, the continuation of affirmative action in higher education, the maintenance of tribal sovereignty, and the ability of state courts to check efforts by state legislatures to gerrymander or even ignore the voters' will in federal elections.

Other important cases relating to firearm regulations, abortion access, and the Affordable Care Act may come from the court's so-called "shadow docket" that deals with emergency petitions. Although the outlook for health before the current deeply conservative Supreme Court majority does not seem propitious, Wiley notes that the "legal landscape" is "changing rapidly" and today's health-harming decisions may not have long legs. To facilitate the short reign of these decisions, she calls on dissenting jurists and legal commentators to "lay the groundwork for more just approaches in the future."

Gostin's editorial (p. 272) concludes this special section. Although his initial focus is on the article authored by Parmet and Khalik, Gostin's piece serves as a coda to the section's main themes, emphasizing how judicial decisions have undercut the ability of federal administrative agencies to protect health. The Supreme Court's decision to block the CDC's eviction moratorium, as described by Parmet and Khalik, is an example of how the court has used the "major questions" doctrine during the pandemic to limit administrative agency actions that may have major economic or political impact to those with explicit statutory authority. Moreover, the application of this approach may extend beyond health emergencies to more "settled" areas of law, including the Clean Water Act, which the court will consider in the upcoming term.

Gostin also reminds us that, although science matters in helping to shield against uninformed legal challenges, ultimately courts are more likely to rule in the direction of what the public views as favorable. Has there ever been a more critical period for a well-informed citizenry? AJPH

CORRESPONDENCE

Correspondence should be sent to Paul C. Erwin, MD, DrPH, Dean and Professor, School of Public Health, University of Alabama at Birmingham, 1665 University Blvd, RPHB 140B, Birmingham, AL 35294-0022 (e-mail: perwin@uab.edu, 205-934-9416). Reprints can be ordered at http://www.ajph.org by clicking the "Reprints" link.

PUBLICATION INFORMATION

Full Citation: Parmet WE, Erwin PC. The challenges to public health law in the aftermath of COVID-19. *Am J Public Health*. 2023;113(3):267–268.

Acceptance Date: December 20, 2022.

DOI: https://doi.org/10.2105/AJPH.2022.307208

CONTRIBUTORS

Both authors participated fully in drafting the editorial and in subsequent writing, editing, and revising.

CONFLICTS OF INTEREST

The authors have no conflicts of interest to disclose.

REFERENCES

1. Bent Weber S, Pepin D. Why law is a determinant of health. *Stetson Law Rev*. 2020;50:401.
2. Borjas GJ. Business closures, stay-at-home restrictions, and COVID-19 testing outcomes in New York City. *Prev Chronic Dis*. 2020;17:E109. https://doi.org/10.5888/pcd17.200264
3. Aylward J, Laderman E, Oliveira LE, Teng G. How much did the CARES Act help households stay afloat? Available at: https://www.frbsf.org/wp-content/uploads/sites/4/el2021-18.pdf. Accessed October 20, 2022.
4. Parmet WE, Burris S, Gable L, de Guia S, Levin DE, Terry NP. COVID-19: the promise and failure of law in an inequitable nation. *Am J Public Health*. 2021;111(1):47–49. https://doi.org/10.2105/AJPH.2020.306008

The 2023 US Supreme Court Term: Implications for Public Health

Lindsay F. Wiley, JD, MPH

ABOUT THE AUTHOR

Lindsay F. Wiley, JD, MPH, is with the University of California, Los Angeles School of Law.

See also Parmet and Erwin, p. 267, Gostin, p. 272, Hodge et al., p. 275, Parmet and Khalik, p. 280, and Platt et al., p. 288.

The US Supreme Court's 2023 term will have important implications for public health, equity, and the power of communities to create healthier living conditions.[1] For the second year in a row, the Court has granted review in cases in which the results would previously have been considered obvious under settled law. The majority's choice to take these cases up may signal that more precedent-refuting decisions are in the offing.

This year, the focus is on the rights of Medicaid beneficiaries, freedom of expression, equal protection, tribal sovereignty, and voting rights. The health consequences of the Court's decisions this year may be less direct and less dramatic than those triggered by *Dobbs v. Jackson Women's Health Organization* (ending federal constitutional protection for reproductive freedom)[2] and *New York State Rifle and Pistol Association v Bruen* (expanding the right to bear arms) in 2022.[3] The questions the Court has taken up for 2023 are more technical, and the majority's decisions may be more nuanced, making it harder to convey to the public how high the stakes are.

THE RIGHTS OF MEDICAID BENEFICIARIES

The case with the most direct relevance to public health invites the Court to block individuals from suing state officials to enforce requirements that attach to federal spending programs. In *Health and Hospital Corporation of Marion County v Talevski*,[4] a patient's family has sued nursing facility administrators for damages arising from violations of Medicaid quality-of-care standards. The nursing home administrators argue that Medicaid is like a contract between states and the federal government, reasoning that enrollees and providers must rely on federal officials to vindicate their interests. If the *Talevski* decision leaves enforcement entirely in the hands of federal officials with limited capacity, it will weaken protection for Medicaid beneficiaries and the safety-net providers who serve them, including provisions related to enrollment, benefits, and choice of providers. It may also have an impact on other federally funded, state-administered programs like the Children's Health Insurance Program and the Supplemental Nutrition Assistance Program.

FREEDOM OF EXPRESSION AS A SHIELD FOR DISCRIMINATION

In *303 Creative v Elenis*,[5] the Court will consider the extent to which commercial activity constitutes constitutionally protected expression that trumps laws prohibiting discrimination by businesses that hold themselves out as offering services to the general public. A for-profit business that designs Web sites is asserting its right to discriminate against same-sex couples seeking assistance with wedding Web sites. The case has implications for efforts to protect lesbian, gay, bisexual, transgender, queer, or questioning people and other groups from discrimination, stigmatization, and associated health harms by limiting the reach of civil rights laws. More broadly, characterization of an expanded range of commercial activity as "expression" that triggers strict scrutiny of government intervention could have implications for efforts to regulate the commercial determinants of health. It could lay the groundwork for businesses to assert that the prices they charge, the products they sell, and the configurations in which they sell them are forms of expression protected from regulation.

EQUAL PROTECTION, DIVERSITY, AND ANTISUBORDINATION

The Court is also hearing cases on whether race-conscious college admissions (*Students for Fair Admissions v Harvard College* and *Students for Fair*

AJPH March 2023, Vol 113, No. 3

Admissions v UNC[6]) and preferences for placing children who are eligible to be members of Indian Tribes with families who are also members (*Brackeen v Haaland*[7]) violate the Constitution's guarantee of equal protection under law. The Supreme Court majority has indicated a preference for race-blind policies and could use the Equal Protection Clause as a basis for invalidating programs that draw distinctions based on race, ethnicity, or tribal membership for the purposes of providing benefits to historically subordinated groups and increasing diversity, equity, and inclusion. Ending race-conscious admissions could have dire consequences for efforts to create a more diverse health workforce, with resulting impacts on quality of care and on who is at the table in discussions about equity in public health. A decision treating "Indian" as a racial classification, rather than a political classification, would call into question programs that protect tribal members from violence and provide them with health benefits.

TRIBAL SOVEREIGNTY AND SELF-DETERMINATION

In addition to challenging the Indian Child Welfare Act on the grounds that it impermissibly discriminates on the basis of race, *Brackeen v. Haaland* raises the possibility that the Supreme Court could further erode tribal sovereignty. Tribal sovereignty and self-determination have important implications for public health, as indicated by recent clashes between tribes and state governors who sought to reverse COVID-19 mitigation measures and anticipated conflicts over reproductive health.[8]

ELECTION LAW AND THE FUTURE OF DEMOCRATIC GOVERNANCE

Moore v Harper[9] is likely to be the most closely watched decision of the term because of its importance to the future of democratic governance. The petitioners are challenging a decision by the North Carolina Supreme Court rejecting a politically gerrymandered election map, which by itself might be unremarkable. Their reliance on the controversial "independent state legislature" theory raises the stakes. If the US Supreme Court were to accept the petitioners' argument that state courts are prohibited by the federal Constitution from reviewing election rules adopted by state legislatures, the decision could pave the way for state legislatures to revamp elections in a host of ways that favor the political party in power. Democratic governance is vital to ensure communities are empowered to create the conditions required for people to be healthy. Giving state legislators carte blanche to set redistricting and election rules with virtually no checks and balances could disempower communities and exacerbate distrust of government as a mechanism for collective action to improve health.

WATCHING THE SHADOW DOCKET

In addition to the cases that are already on the docket, the Court is also likely to continue its trend of intervening more actively via the expedited and less transparent process of the so-called "shadow docket."[10] The Court could grant review in several additional cases with major public health implications. The lower federal courts are still grappling with the fallout from the Supreme Court's blockbuster 2021 and 2022 terms. The environment is dynamic and highly partisan, and the Court could take up a question presented by ongoing litigation on a moment's notice.

For example, several recent lower court decisions have invalidated longstanding gun-control regulations under the new "history and tradition" standard adopted in *Bruen*.[11] Complex abortion issues are emerging in the aftermath of *Dobbs*.[12] For example, lower courts are split over whether federal health law preempts criminalization of pregnancy termination when necessary to stabilize an emergency medical condition.[13] Lower courts are also split over whether the Supreme Court's new approach to religious liberty means that refusal of religious exemptions from government vaccination requirements triggers strict scrutiny.[14] In addition, some lower court judges—perhaps emboldened by the Court's willingness to abandon precedents it disagrees with on ideological grounds—are pushing fringe ideas into the mainstream, offering them up for the new majority's consideration. For example, a case making its way up through the lower courts could unwind the Affordable Care Act's requirement to cover preventive services with no out-of-pocket costs.[15]

ENVISIONING A MORE JUST FUTURE IN A TIME OF RADICAL RETRENCHMENT

The legal landscape public health interventions must navigate is changing rapidly. The analysis of the current majority of the Court may ultimately make it easier for a future majority to reverse recent decisions. The conservative legal movement has played a long game to achieve dramatic reversals of the precedents that stood in the way of their ideological goals. Dissenting justices and legal commentators play an important role by documenting the inaccuracies of the current majority's analysis and laying the groundwork for more just approaches in the future. AJPH

CORRESPONDENCE

Correspondence should be sent to Lindsay F. Wiley, UCLA School of Law, 385 Charles E Young Dr E, Los Angeles, CA 90095 (e-mail: wiley@law.ucla.edu). Reprints can be ordered at https://ajph.org by clicking the "Reprints" link.

PUBLICATION INFORMATION

Full Citation: Wiley LF. The 2023 US supreme court term: implications for public health. *Am J Public Health*. 2023;113(3):269–271.

Acceptance Date: December 18, 2022.

DOI: https://doi.org/10.2105/AJPH.2022.307210

CONFLICTS OF INTEREST

The author has no conflicts of interest to disclose.

REFERENCES

1. Williams MA, Gostin LO. Will there be a Supreme assault on public health? *STAT.* October 3, 2022. Available at: https://www.statnews.com/2022/10/03/will-there-be-a-supreme-court-assault-on-public-health. Accessed December 8, 2022.
2. *Dobbs v Jackson Women's Health Organization*, 142 SCt 2228 (2022).
3. *New York State Rifle and Pistol Association v Bruen*, 142 SCt 2111 (2022).
4. Rudowitz R, Sobel L. What is at stake for Medicaid in Supreme Court Case Health & Hospital Corp v. Talevski? *KFF Policy Watch.* October 28, 2022. Available at: https://www.kff.org/policy-watch/what-is-at-stake-for-medicaid-in-supreme-court-case-health-hospital-corp-v-talevski. Accessed December 8, 2022.
5. Keren H. The alarming legal strategy behind a SCOTUS case that could undo decades of civil rights protections. *Slate.* March 9, 2022. Available at: https://slate.com/news-and-politics/2022/03/supreme-court-303-creative-coordinated-anti-lgbt-legal-strategy.html. Accessed December 8, 2022.
6. Hodge JG. Affirmative action and public health repercussions. Network for Public Health Law. November 23, 2022. Available at: https://www.networkforphl.org/resources/affirmative-action-and-public-health-repercussions. Accessed December 8, 2022.
7. National Council of Urban Indian Health signs on to amicus brief in support of the Indian Child Welfare Act. September 9, 2022. Available at: https://indiancountrytoday.com/the-press-pool/national-council-of-urban-indian-health-signs-on-to-amicus-brief-in-support-of-the-indian-child-welfare-act. Accessed December 8, 2022.
8. Hoss A. Toward Tribal health sovereignty. *Wisconsin Law Review.* 2022;(2):413–442.
9. Savitzky A. and Graunke K. Explaining Moore v. Harper, the Supreme Court case that could upend democracy. ACLU. December 6, 2022. Available at: https://www.aclu.org/news/voting-rights/explaining-moore-v-harper-the-supreme-court-case-that-could-upend-democracy. Accessed December 8, 2022.
10. Vladeck S. "Shadow dockets" are normal. The way SCOTUS is using them is the problem. *Slate.* April 12, 2021. Available at: https://slate.com/news-and-politics/2021/04/scotus-shadow-docket-use-problem.html. Accessed December 8, 2022.
11. Charles J. Worrying trends in the lower courts after Bruen. Duke Center for Firearms Law. September 30, 2022. Available at: https://firearmslaw.duke.edu/2022/09/worrying-trends-in-the-lower-courts-after-bruen. Accessed December 8, 2022.
12. Cohen DS, Donley G, Rebouché R. The new abortion battleground. *Columbia Law Review.* August 30, 2022. Available at: https://papers.ssrn.com/sol3/papers.cfm?abstract_id=4032931. Accessed December 8, 2022.
13. American Health Law Association. Courts split on whether EMTALA preempts state abortion ban laws. *Health Law Weekly.* August 26, 2022. Available at: https://www.americanhealthlaw.org/content-library/health-law-weekly/article/5e14aee8-db53-4517-8579-7f818cdaa9ea/Courts-Split-on-Whether-EMTALA-Preempts-State-Abor. Accessed December 8, 2022.
14. *Doster v Kendall*, 22-3497/3702 (6th Cir 2022).
15. *Braidwood Management v Becerra*, Civil Action 4:20-cv-00283-O (ND Tex 2022).

Judicial Trends in the Era of COVID-19: Public Health in Peril

Lawrence O. Gostin, JD, LLD

ABOUT THE AUTHOR

Lawrence O. Gostin is Founding O'Neill Professor of Global Health Law and Faculty Director of the O'Neill Institute at Georgetown University, Washington, DC. He directs the World Health Organization Collaborating Center on National and Global Health Law and sits on the WHO Review Committee to Revise the International Health Regulations in light of the COVID-19 pandemic.

See also Parmet and Erwin, p. 267, Wiley, p. 269, Hodge et al., p. 275, Parmet and Khalik, p. 280, and Platt et al., p. 288.

AJPH March 2023, Vol 113, No. 3

A pandemic can test and reshape health systems like no other event. The same can be said for the profound impacts of pandemics on public health law and governance. January 2023 marks the third anniversary of COVID-19. As the pandemic wrought devastation on health and the economy, public health officials exercised unprecedented powers, ranging from orders to mask, test, and vaccinate to social distancing, school and business closures, and stay-at-home orders. These powers unleashed an avalanche of legal challenges to curb emergency health powers and agencies' ability to safeguard the public's health and safety.

In this issue of *AJPH*, Parmet and Khalik (p. 280) provide a majestic analysis of judicial litigation during the COVID-19 pandemic, demonstrating the judiciary's outsized role. Their article shines a light into a modern judicial era where judges substitute their judgment for that of career scientists. Parmet and Khalik also offer important insights on how to shape policies to withstand aggressive judicial scrutiny.

Donald Trump appointed one third of the US Supreme Court (now with a 6–3 conservative supermajority) and 30% of all federal appellate judges.[1] Many are hewing to the political ideologies of their appointing president, often closely tracking far-right policies. Litigators "forum shop" to get their cases in front of judges sympathetic to their cause. Consider how a single federal judge in Florida, a Trump appointee rated "unqualified" by the American Bar Association, was able to nationally block the Centers for Disease Control and Prevention's (CDC's) transit mask mandate in April 2022.[2]

Parmet and Khalik analyzed over 1000 federal and state judicial decisions opining on the lawfulness of public health powers during the COVID-19 pandemic. Although over three fourths of those decisions upheld pandemic orders, courts often gave precedence to personal and religious freedoms over public health powers. In high-profile cases, the Supreme Court has dangerously narrowed the scope of administrative agencies' rule-making powers—and that trend is only likely to accelerate in the court's 2023 term.

RIGHTS-BASED CHALLENGES TO PUBLIC HEALTH MEASURES

In the landmark 1905 ruling *Jacobson v Massachusetts*, Justice Harlan famously stated, "The liberty secured by the Constitution to every person does not import an absolute right in each person to be, at all times and in all circumstances, wholly freed from restraint. There are manifold restraints to which every person is necessarily subject for the common good."[3] Throughout the COVID-19 pandemic, courts largely upheld state and municipal measures to protect the common good.

However, as Parmet and Khalik's research revealed, legal challenges to COVID-19 containment measures were most often successful when grounded in religious freedoms. Conservative courts are viewing religious freedom as a near-absolute right—a dangerous trend that could weaken public health.[4] Consider how the Supreme Court repeatedly rejected religious challenges to restrictions on gatherings with a narrow five to four majority. When Amy Coney Barrett replaced Ruth Bader Ginsburg in October 2020, the court abruptly reversed itself, all but ignoring its recent precedents. The court struck down gathering restrictions in New York[5] and California,[6] designed to mitigate COVID-19 mass spreading events—ignoring a history of mass spreading events at religious congregations.

This could just be the beginning of courts jeopardizing public health powers in the name of religious freedom. In a concurring opinion last term, Justice Alito urged overturning *Employment Division v Smith*, which ruled that individuals cannot disobey general health and safety rules for religious reasons.[7] Overturning this precedent would open the door to vast discrimination in the name of religion, contributing to physical and psychological health harms and widening health inequities. Further, as Parmet and Khalik point out, the Supreme Court's stance on religion could undermine state vaccine mandates that fail to provide broad religious exemptions. Vaccine-preventable childhood diseases like measles often occur in geographic areas with high rates of unvaccinated individuals, principally in religious communities.[8]

REGULATORY AUTHORITY OF EXECUTIVE AGENCIES

Administrative agencies provide a web of protection for health, safety, and the environment. Agencies are staffed with career professionals who can evaluate evolving scientific standards, while acting far more rapidly and flexibly than a legislature. Legislatures have thus delegated wide rule-making powers to agencies to curtail threats to health and the environment. Since Franklin Delano Roosevelt, courts have granted considerable deference to executive discretion. Ignoring long-standing precedent, the Supreme Court, as well as lower courts, have begun to rein in executive action, arguing that legislatures had not explicitly authorized the action. Parmet and Khalik identify a dangerous trend: courts were most likely to weigh in and overturn executive action in "purple states"—that is, those with a Democratic governor and a Republican-majority legislature. This finding makes it ever clearer that courts are putting partisan politics ahead of public health.

The Supreme Court has similarly narrowed the scope of what federal agencies can do, such as by blocking the CDC's housing eviction moratorium using the "major questions" doctrine, which provides that any administrative measure of broad economic or political significance must be backed by explicit statutory authority. Until recently, this doctrine never captured a majority of justices; today, it is a conservative highway for striking down agency actions. In a concurrence to *National Federation of Independent Business v Department of Labor* (in which the Supreme Court invalidated an Occupational Safety and Health Administration [OSHA] emergency measure requiring COVID-19 vaccination or weekly testing for large employers),[9] three justices (Gorsuch, Alito, and Thomas) advocated for the major questions doctrine. In *West Virginia v Environmental Protection Agency* (EPA), Justice Robert's majority opinion, joined by the five other conservative justices, relied on the major questions doctrine to hold the EPA's emissions rules for protecting against harmful pollutants unconstitutional.[10] Next term, the court will weigh in on the Clean Water Act, with a sadly all-too-predictable outcome of further narrowing health and safety powers.

When the next major health emergency strikes, we may begin to fully understand the ramifications of weakening agencies' authority to meet health and environmental challenges while protecting the most vulnerable.

NAVIGATING THE RESTORATION OF PUBLIC HEALTH AUTHORITY

Given these judicial trends, how can we secure the future of public health law and policy? Creating a more balanced, less partisan federal court system would require key reforms. Yet judicial reforms will require significant time and political will, so policymakers need to be able to operate effectively in the environment that we find ourselves in.

Grounding public health measures in science is especially important, as sound scientific evidence could help shield against legal challenges. Scientific assessments, of course, are challenging during health emergencies when the evidence is uncertain and evolving. (Think back to the early days of the COVID-19 pandemic on issues like masking and aerosolized spread.) Scientists and lawmakers alike must be clear on what they know and what they don't know, and communicate transparently to gain public trust. As Parmet and Khalik observe, it may be more difficult for a judge to overturn a law or regulation that the public views favorably.

Lawmakers must also be cognizant of the possible impact of public health measures on the exercise of religion that could lead to legal and constitutional challenges. Religious groups must not become the enemy of public health; instead, policymakers should engage smartly with religious and community leaders, whom the public often holds in high regard. Finding common ground and engaging with diverse religious and political constituencies could potentially reduce opposition to public health measures.

When it comes to safeguarding the public against immediate and serious threats to public health, Parmet and Khalik speak compellingly. Public health officials "should not be dissuaded from issuing critical orders or regulations because of overblown fears of litigation." To do so would be an abdication of the responsibility to act for the common good. Rather, when acting at the height of their powers, public health officials must anticipate litigation and be prepared to answer foreseeable challenges.

The COVID-19 pandemic seemed to unravel so many communal bonds of shared and mutual responsibilities to take care of one another. This splintering of the social fabric manifested in the political branches of government as well as in the judiciary. To avoid a future disaster of the magnitude of COVID-19 (or even worse), we have to find ways to come together, support science, and grant public health officials scope to act for the public welfare. AJPH

CORRESPONDENCE

Correspondence should be sent to Lawrence O. Gostin, JD, LLD, O'Neill Institute for National and Global Health Law, Georgetown University Law Center, 600 New Jersey Ave NW, Washington, DC 20001 (gostin@georgetown.edu). Reprints can be ordered at http://www.ajph.org by clicking the "Reprints" link.

PUBLICATION INFORMATION

Full Citation: Gostin LO. Judicial trends in the era of COVID-19: public health in peril. *Am J Public Health*. 2023;113(3):272–274.

Acceptance Date: December 15, 2022.

DOI: https://doi.org/10.2105/AJPH.2022.307211

CONFLICTS OF INTEREST

The author has no conflicts of interest to declare.

REFERENCES

1. Scheindlin SA. Trump's judges will call the shots for years to come. The judicial system is broken. *The Guardian*. October 25, 2021. Available at: https://www.theguardian.com/commentisfree/2021/oct/25/trump-judges-supreme-court-justices-judiciary. Accessed January 17, 2023.
2. Gostin LO, Hosie D. No matter how you feel about masks, you should be alarmed by this judge's decision. *New York Times*. April 25, 2022. Available at: https://www.nytimes.com/2022/04/25/opinion/masks-covid-ban.html?referringSource=articleShare. Accessed January 17, 2023.
3. *Jacobson v Massachusetts*, 197 US 11 (1905).
4. Gostin LO. The Supreme Court's new majority threatens 155 years of deference to public officials handling public health emergencies. *Forbes*. December 11, 2020. Available at: https://www.forbes.com/sites/coronavirusfrontlines/2020/12/11/the-supreme-courts-new-majority-threatens-115-years-of-deference-to-public-officials-handling-health-emergencies/?sh=205025283a4b. Accessed January 17, 2023.
5. *Roman Catholic Diocese of Brooklyn, New York v Cuomo*, 592 US _ (2020).
6. *Tandon v Newsom*, 593 US _ (2021).
7. *Employment Division v Smith*, 494 US 872 (1990).
8. Sinclair DR, Grefenstette JJ, Krauland MG, et al. Forecasted size of measles outbreaks associated with vaccination exemptions for schoolchildren. *JAMA Netw Open*. 2019;2(8):e199768. https://doi.org/10.1001/jamanetworkopen.2019.9768
9. *National Federation of Independent Business v Department of Labor, Occupational Safety and Health Administration*, 595 US _ (2022).
10. *West Virginia v Environmental Protection Agency*, 597 US __ (2022).

State Public Health Emergency Powers in Response to COVID-19

James G. Hodge Jr., JD, LLM, Lauren T. Dunning, JD, MPH, and Jennifer L. Piatt, JD

ABOUT THE AUTHORS

James G. Hodge Jr. and Jennifer L. Piatt are with the Center for Public Health Law and Policy, Sandra Day O'Connor College of Law, Arizona State University, Phoenix, AZ. Lauren T. Dunning is with the Milken Institute Center for the Future of Aging, Santa Monica, CA.

See also Parmet and Erwin, p. 267, Wiley, p. 269, Gostin, p. 272, Parmet and Khalik, p. 280, and Platt et al., p. 288.

The September 11 terrorist attacks and the anthrax exposures in fall 2001 changed perceptions of emergency risks in the United States, igniting an era of intense preparedness and response undergirded by substantial funding, interjurisdictional efforts, and comprehensive, state-based legal reforms. Over ensuing years, states infused "public health emergency" (PHE) declarations and powers to test, screen, separate, treat, survey, and vaccinate individuals and groups into their laws on the basis, in large part, of the foundational Model State Emergency Health Powers Act (MSEHPA) finalized in December 2001.[1] Initial PHE declarations and limited exercises of these powers among select states emerged in response to infectious disease outbreaks including the H1N1, Ebola, and Zika viruses.

None of these threats, however, rivals COVID-19. With 630 million reported infections globally and more than a million confirmed US deaths in 2.9 years,[2] the pandemic warranted "all-stops" efforts. Every state declared some type of emergency in the first 10 weeks of the pandemic in early 2020.[1] Widespread implementation of social distancing requirements—isolation, quarantine, closures, travel restrictions, stay-at-home orders—unquestionably saved lives but also carried substantial societal costs.[3]

Public reactions to expansive use of PHE powers were fierce. The pandemic was rapidly politicized. A tsunami of litigation flooded courts nationally.[3] Voters confronted governors and public health officials. Presidential administrations changed mid-pandemic. As the epidemiology of COVID-19 became clearer and safe, efficacious vaccines were developed and distributed, applications of state PHE laws and policies oscillated over multiple waves of infections. Uses of these powers were shaped by "denialist" laws and policies (expressly rejecting known and actual public health risks), federal shifts in responses, and judicial restraints based on misperceptions of individual rights and structural limits underlying governmental responses.[4] We explore these themes here through assessments of core legal foundations for modern state emergency powers, their uses and challenges in response to COVID-19, and postpandemic reform proposals to improve state responses to future emergency threats.

LEGAL FOUNDATIONS OF EMERGENCY HEALTH POWERS

Federal emergency preparedness and response laws are limited to appropriate exercises of constitutionally enumerated powers (e.g., to tax and spend, regulate interstate commerce, or protect national security). So long as federal laws are constitutionally crafted, they are supreme over state and local laws. Conversely, states are reserved broad "police powers" to provide for the health, safety, morals, and general welfare of populations as per the Constitution's Tenth Amendment. Pursuant to these authorities, states have crafted varied responses to an extensive array of threats (e.g., hurricanes, fires, floods, chemical releases, attacks, epidemics) through legal declarations of emergencies or disasters reflecting an "all-hazards approach."[1]

The 2001 terrorist and bioterrorism attacks led to modernization of a patchwork of inconsistent and incongruous state emergency laws through the development of MSEHPA in fall 2001. Drafters of the act clearly distinguished health crises from other extant emergencies. A public health emergency was defined as "an occurrence or imminent threat of an illness or health condition" (stemming from bioterrorism, emerging infectious diseases, or other causes) posing a substantial risk of significant deaths, disabilities, or future health harms.[1(p376)] Emergency responses authorized via gubernatorial declarations of a PHE, as per MSEHPA section 601, broadly included use of all available means to limit infectious disease

AJPH March 2022, Vol 113, No. 3

transmissions and ensure that contagious cases are subject to proper control and treatment.

Unlike most existing state emergency laws, however, MSEHPA drafters also provided a comprehensive menu of provisions to detect and manage PHEs. As shown in Table 1, these provisions included expedited public health powers related to individuals (e.g., testing, vaccination, isolation, quarantine), entities (e.g., inspection, closure, evacuation), and private property (e.g., nuisance abatement). Subject to scholarly debate,[5] these PHE measures were balanced in the act with express due process and other safeguards designed to protect civil liberties from governmental overreach. By 2006, 38 states had adopted various MSEHPA provisions through state legislation or regulatory reforms. In turn, these laws were selectively used in response to emerging viral diseases (e.g., H1N1 [2009/2010], Ebola [2015], and Zika [2018]) and other noninfectious public health threats (e.g., opioid use disorder, natural disasters, racism).[6]

USE OF EMERGENCY HEALTH POWERS DURING COVID-19

Limited exercises of state PHE powers, however, could not approximate the widescale, national implementation of responses to COVID-19. After early signs of a potentially deadly new strain of coronavirus emerged globally in late 2019, index COVID-19 cases were detected in the United States beginning in January 2020.[7] Real-time public health responses quickly followed. On January 31, Department of Health and Human Services secretary Alex Azar declared a national PHE, followed by President Trump's emergency declarations on March 13, 2020.[1] By the end of March, emergencies of all types had been declared across all 50 states, a first in US history.[8] Despite widespread adoption of MSEHPA provisions, only 13 states formally declared PHEs. Four states (Florida, Maryland, New Jersey, and Ohio) declared PHEs in combination with general emergencies.[8] Most other states relied on the aforementioned "all-hazards" declarations of emergencies (33 states) or disasters (four states) to effectuate their responses.[8]

Multifarious practical, legal, and political reasons help explain the diversity of state-based declarations according to information garnered by the Network for Public Health Law and its national partners assisting public health actors during the COVID-19 pandemic. The sheer enormity of logistics challenges posed by the pandemic (e.g., managing patient surges, ensuring continued hospital operations, addressing supply

TABLE 1— MSEHPA Key Subjects and Provisions

Subject	Key Provisions
Planning for PHEs	Establishes a state-level PHE planning commission Requires a PHE plan detailing provisions for coordination of response resources and services across agencies Sets guidelines to carry out specific actions such as testing and treatment
Detecting and tracking PHEs	Establishes reporting of illnesses and health conditions that may cause a PHE and prescription patterns indicating a potential PHE Requires public health agencies to ascertain potential causes of a PHE Empowers agencies to investigate cases, identify exposed individuals, and implement control measures
Declaring PHEs	Enables a governor to declare a PHE, typically after consultation with public health experts Authorizes emergency powers to use and mobilize state resources and seek aid from the federal government and other states Allows for termination of a PHE, including by declaration of the governor, majority vote of the legislature, or automatically after 30 days (if not renewed)
Managing property	Authorizes public health agencies to close, evacuate, and decontaminate facilities and materials Empowers public health agencies to use private materials and facilities to respond to the PHE, control public roads and areas, and regulate the use and sale of necessities (e.g., food, fuel, health care supplies) Controls the disposal of infectious waste and safe handling of human remains
Protecting individuals	Enables public health agencies to medically examine, test, vaccinate, and treat individuals subject to limitations Authorizes isolation and quarantine of individuals or groups to prevent the spread of contagious diseases through the least restrictive means available Reciprocates licensure for out-of-state health care personnel
Providing information and immunity	Requires public health agencies to share information regarding a PHE through culturally respectful and accessible communications Provides immunity for state and local actors responding to a PHE Insulates health care workers and other private actors or entities from liability for noncriminal acts in response to a PHE

Note. MSEHPA = Model State Emergency Health Powers Act; PHE = public health emergency.

chain interruptions) led some governors to seek a wider array of emergency powers through general declarations. Use of executive waiver authorities pursuant to emergency or disaster declarations enabled governors to selectively and temporarily set aside legislative or other nonconstitutional requirements inhibiting governmental response efforts (e.g., state-based procurement laws regarding agency purchases of needed supplies).

Broader legal options available under general emergency declarations facilitated executive branch efforts to address economic effects (e.g., temporary closures, job losses, unemployment claims) of the pandemic. Leaders declared emergencies to trigger statewide emergency operations plans, launch incident command systems, invoke intrastate mobilization agreements, or facilitate exchange of resources across state borders through the Emergency Management Assistance Compact. Some governors viewed emergency or disaster declarations as necessary to pursue expense reimbursements through the Federal Emergency Management Agency or receive direct federal assistance through the Department of Health and Human Services and other agencies. From a political perspective, emergency or disaster declarations may have heightened awareness among state populations of the immense risks posed by the pandemic.

Irrespective of the type of declaration, state governors and officials wielded emergency powers to issue numerous orders in the first 90 days of the pandemic clarifying public health responses via statutory or regulatory emergency provisions assimilating MSEHPA authorities (Table 1).[8] Testing, screening, reporting, and surveillance efforts were activated. Initial cases were assessed through contact tracing. As epidemiologists surmised the stealthy nature of asymptomatic COVID-19 infections, creating distance among US residents became a central public health strategy.[3] Mask requirements, shunned initially, were later instituted in many public settings for months on end. Widespread use of quarantine and isolation powers affected tens of thousands of residents. Most people voluntarily complied with measures consistent with model MSEHPA policies, but some recalcitrants faced more forceful interventions or penalties.[1]

Across the nation, nonessential businesses, religious institutions, and schools were closed beginning in spring 2020. Health care providers facing patient surges shut off access to visitors. Group assembly limits were implemented, including nightly curfews in select jurisdictions.[3] Travel restrictions and limited border closures were instituted. Forty-five states issued stay-at-home orders for weeks beginning in late March 2020 through general emergency powers, including MSEHPA section 601.[8] Work, school, and social activities were halted or shifted to virtual formats as people awaited safe, effective vaccines. Although residents' tolerance for extreme social distancing quickly waned as the effects of long-term separations mounted, initial implementation of these measures prevented countless infections and saved lives.[9]

CHANGING DYNAMICS AND LEGAL CHALLENGES

At the onset of the pandemic, President Trump deferred to states' frontline responses,[10] focusing national efforts instead on vaccine development and production. Lacking federal leadership, state-based COVID-19 response efforts quickly diverged as legal and political objections arose. Through extensive judicial challenges, complainants argued that public health mitigation measures infringed on individual liberties, including freedoms of speech and association, religious liberty, rights to due process or bear arms, and equal protections.[3]

MSEHPA drafters had expressly stipulated that individual rights should be respected to the extent possible when implementing specific measures (e.g., requiring use of least restrictive means regarding isolation or quarantine).[1] Despite long-standing constitutional recognition of the need to balance individual liberties with communal health needs, claimants asserted that their constitutionally protected interests predominated over public health. Litigation over the scope of PHE powers was spearheaded by multiple US Supreme Court decisions striking down COVID-19 assembly restrictions affecting religious entities (November 2020) and deauthorizing the Centers for Disease Control and Prevention's national residential eviction moratorium (August 2021).[1]

Judicial cases also raised structural arguments centered on separation of powers,[1] preemption, and local "home rule" authorities.[11] In May 2020, Wisconsin's supreme court overturned the COVID-19 PHE order of the state's health department.[12] The court determined that the department failed to follow procedural rules in promulgating the order as a regulation pursuant to Wisconsin's statutory definition of "rule."[12] Rigid judicial interpretations limiting executive PHE powers diminished state and local health agencies' authorities in other states including Georgia, Kentucky, Michigan, and Ohio.

Federal public health powers were similarly debated. On January 13, 2022, the US Supreme Court renounced the authority of the Occupational Safety and Health Administration to require large businesses to impose vaccine-or-test requirements on employees[13] while allowing a similar mandate affecting health care workers set by the Centers for Medicare & Medicaid Services. In April 2022, a federal district court struck down the Centers for Disease Control and Prevention's authority to issue its mass transportation mask order,[14] leading multiple states to drop their requirements.

Politics contributed to temporary implementations or premature rescissions of emergency declarations, stay-at-home orders, and other interventions.[15] Extreme politicization led multiple states to limit or cease emergency authorities, vaccination and mask mandates, and social distancing efforts in furtherance of protecting individual freedoms and promoting economic interests. The public health consequences of these actions were immense. Failure to implement vaccine mandates or passport requirements (e.g., checking vaccination status for entry into specific public settings) inhibited immunization rates. School districts without universal masking protocols experienced elevated numbers of COVID-19 cases.[16] One assessment of stay-at-home orders demonstrated faster declining COVID-19 case rates in 2647 counties implementing such orders in comparison with 368 counties without them over a three-week period in 2020.[17]

States' conservative approaches to public health prevention and response led to excess COVID-19 cases and deaths overall. From June 3 to December 13, 2020, case and death counts in 26 states with Republican governors were up to 1.8 times higher per 100 000 residents than 25 states (and the District of Columbia) with Democratic leaders.[15] Ultimately, thousands died from COVID-19 because their governments refused to employ proven, preventive measures. US life expectancy plunged by more than two years from the start of the pandemic to 2022.[18]

State legislative and regulatory responses also had an impact. A bevy of statutes and regulations across at least half of the states explicitly sought to curb public health powers in response to COVID-19, other health emergencies, and even in routine settings. Although the threat of denialist state laws was palpable, legal counter-efforts surfaced as well, especially related to mask requirements.

Legislative or gubernatorial efforts to rescind school mask mandates in Arizona and Texas in 2021 were initially dismissed by courts on constitutional or procedural grounds.[4] When Arizona governor Doug Ducey attempted on August 17, 2021, to deny federal response funds to school districts imposing mask requirements, the US Department of the Treasury rejected his authority to do so.[4] That same day, federal Department of Education secretary Miguel Cardona announced legal actions to counter mask bans including challenges under the Americans with Disabilities Act.[4] After the Michigan supreme court limited Governor Gretchen Whitmer's emergency authorities in October 2020, the state health department pivoted to order face coverings in schools through its existing routine public health powers.[4]

REFORM EFFORTS TO ENHANCE STATE PUBLIC HEALTH POWERS

A resounding legal takeaway from the COVID-19 pandemic is the continued need for clarity and consistency of authorized governmental actions when US residents' lives are at stake. Future coordinated federal responses may help resolve conflicting exercises of state PHE powers,[4] but state-level public health interventions remain essential to effective emergency responses in our federalist system. Shortcomings of state responses to COVID-19, legislative and judicial challenges to public health powers, and discordance over levels of governmental authority warrant ongoing assessments and efforts to bolster state PHE response capacities. Emerging disease outbreaks arising from new strains of COVID-19, monkeypox, measles, polio, Marburg virus, and other globally circulating conditions present extant threats substantiating real-time legal reforms.

Even as multiple states sought to limit PHE authorities during the pandemic through denialist laws and policies, other state legislatures introduced laws to reinforce health infrastructure or enhance public health powers[19] through the following strategies:

1. Creating advisory bodies to assess and make recommendations on PHE authorities: Alabama's joint resolution (enacted April 29, 2021) promotes assessments of state COVID-19 responses to generate efficacious policies.[20]
2. Strengthening local public health authority and coordination: Oklahoma Senate Bill 736 (April 27, 2021) enables counties to form health districts sharing resources to improve health outcomes.[21]
3. Increasing transparency and accountability: Colorado's House Bill 1426 (July 14, 2020) requires regular gubernatorial briefings to the legislature in declared emergencies.[22]

State leaders and policymakers are aligning across states to remake the US public health infrastructure postpandemic. A national initiative, Act for Public Health, provides legislative bill tracking, information, and advocacy promoting public health authorities. Select states are reconsidering their powers given adverse judicial treatments and advisory bodies' analyses of COVID-19 responses. A drafting committee of the Uniform Law Commission is producing model language for states on allocation and use of legislative and executive powers in PHEs.[23]

These efforts should be undergirded by commitments to infuse health equity into legal reforms, including emerging PHE legal principles related to compulsory social distancing and allocations of critical medical or other resources pursuant to crisis standards of care.[24] Complementary federal support for uniform response efforts through funding, interstate commerce authorities, and oversight of essential supplies and health services will help recalibrate interjurisdictional responses.[4,11] During the pandemic, for example, states were allowed to use federal funds via the American Rescue Plan Act to incentivize individual vaccinations through direct cash payments, gift cards, lottery programs, and in-kind transfers.[25]

Additional efforts to analyze existing laws and identify solutions across federal and state governments are needed in light of ongoing shifts in constitutional interpretations via the US Supreme Court. Key legal reforms ahead include efforts to (1) clarify the scope and triggers of emergency declarations, (2) refine social distancing and other public health powers, (3) limit denialist political influences, (4) corral rampant misinformation swirling around vaccinations and other public health interventions, and (5) sustain funding for PHE preparedness and response. Rebuilding public health infrastructure and improving health system response capabilities may help ensure that lessons learned from the tragic losses of the COVID-19 pandemic contribute to constructive reforms that alleviate future health threats and promote health equity. AJPH

CORRESPONDENCE

Correspondence should be sent to James G. Hodge Jr., JD, LLM, Sandra Day O'Connor College of Law, Arizona State University, 111 E Taylor St, MC 9520, Phoenix, AZ 85004 (e-mail: james.hodge.1@asu.edu). Reprints can be ordered at http://www.ajph.org by clicking the "Reprints" link.

PUBLICATION INFORMATION

Full Citation: Hodge Jr. JG, Dunning LT, Piatt JL. State public health emergency powers in response to COVID-19. *Am J Public Health*. 2022;113(3): 275–279.

Acceptance Date: October 17, 2022.

DOI: https://doi.org/10.2105/AJPH.2022.307158

CONTRIBUTORS

J. G. Hodge Jr. supervised and contributed to conceptualization, research, and the drafting and editing of the article in all phases. L. T. Dunning and J. L. Piatt contributed to conceptualization, research, and the drafting and editing of the article.

ACKNOWLEDGMENTS

The views expressed are those of the authors and not their institutions.

CONFLICTS OF INTEREST

The authors have no financial, personal, academic, or other conflicts of interest in the subject matter discussed in this article.

REFERENCES

1. Hodge JG. *Public Health Law in a Nutshell*. 4th ed. Eagan, MN: West Academic Publishing; 2021.
2. Johns Hopkins University. Coronavirus resource center. Available at: https://coronavirus.jhu.edu/map.html. Accessed October 31, 2022.
3. Hodge JG, Piatt JL, Carey E, Reinke HN. COVID's constitutional conundrum: assessing individual rights in public health emergencies. *Tenn Law Rev*. 2022;88(1):838–887. https://doi.org/10.2139/ssrn.3802045
4. Hodge JG, Piatt JL, Barraza L. Legal interventions to counter COVID-19 denialism. *J Law Med Ethics*. 2021;49(4):677–682. https://doi.org/10.1017/jme.2021.92
5. Annas GJ. Bioterrorism, public health, and civil liberties. *N Engl J Med*. 2002;346(17):1337–1342. https://doi.org/10.1056/NEJM200204253461722
6. Gostin LO, Nuzzo JB. Twenty years after the anthrax terrorist attacks of 2001: lessons learned and unlearned for the COVID-19 response. *JAMA*. 2021;326(20):2009–2010. https://doi.org/10.1001/jama.2021.19292
7. Holshue ML, DeBolt C, Lindquist S, et al. First case of 2019 novel coronavirus in the United States. *N Engl J Med*. 2020;382(10):929–936. https://doi.org/10.1056/NEJMoa2001191
8. Hodge JG. Emergency legal preparedness: COVID-19. Available at: https://www.networkforphl.org/resources/emergency-legal-preparedness-covid19. Accessed August 25, 2022.
9. Hsiang S, Allen D, Annan-Phan S, et al. The effect of large-scale anti-contagion policies on the COVID-19 pandemic. *Nature*. 2020;584(7820):262–267. https://doi.org/10.1038/s41586-020-2404-8
10. Haffajee RL, Mello MM. Thinking globally, acting locally—the U.S. response to Covid-19. *N Engl J Med*. 2020;382(22):e75. https://doi.org/10.1056/NEJMp2006740
11. Gartner D. Pandemic preemption: limits on local control over public health. Available at: http://nulawreview.org/volume-13-issue-2-articles/gartner. Accessed August 25, 2022.
12. *Wisconsin Legislature v Palm*, 942 NW2d 900 (Wis 2020).
13. *National Federation of Independent Business v Occupational Safety and Health Administration*, 595 US (2022).
14. *Health Freedom Defense Fund, Inc. v Biden*, FSupp 3d (MD Fla 2022).
15. Neelon B, Mutiso F, Mueller NT, et al. Associations between governor political affiliation and COVID-19 cases, deaths, and testing in the U.S. *Am J Prev Med*. 2021;61(1):115–119. https://doi.org/10.1016/j.amepre.2021.01.034
16. Boutzoukas AE, Zimmerman KO, Inkelas M, et al. School masking policies and secondary SARS-CoV-2 transmission. *Pediatrics*. 2022;149(6):e2022056687. https://doi.org/10.1542/peds.2022-056687
17. Fowler JH, Hill SJ, Levin R, Obradovich N. Stay-at-home orders associate with subsequent decreases in COVID-19 cases and fatalities in the United States. *PLoS One*. 2021;16(6):e0248849. https://doi.org/10.1371/journal.pone.0248849
18. Masters RK, Aron LY, Woolf SH. Changes in life expectancy between 2019 and 2021 in the United States and 21 peer countries. *JAMA Netw Open*. 2022;5(4):e227067. https://doi.org/10.1101/2022.04.05.22273393
19. Parmet WE, Burris S, Gable L, et al. COVID-19: the promise and failure of law in an inequitable nation. *Am J Public Health*. 2021;111(1):47–49. https://doi.org/10.2105/AJPH.2020.306008
20. LegiScan. Alabama Senate Joint Resolution 110. Available at: https://legiscan.com/AL/bill/SJR110/2021. Accessed August 25, 2022.
21. LegiScan. Oklahoma Senate Bill 736. Available at: https://legiscan.com/OK/bill/SB736/2021. Accessed August 25, 2022.
22. LegiScan. Colorado House Bill 1426. Available at: https://legiscan.com/CO/bill/HB1426/2020. Accessed August 25, 2022.
23. Uniform Law Commission. Public-Health-Emergency Authority Committee. Available at: https://www.uniformlaws.org/committees/community-home?CommunityKey=be7c4af5-73e0-4307-8d5a-ca281b8216cd. Accessed August 25, 2022.
24. Wiley LF. Democratizing the law of social distancing. *Yale J Health Policy Law Ethics*. 2020;19(3):50–121. https://doi.org/10.2139/ssrn.3634997
25. White House. President Biden to announce new actions to get more Americans vaccinated and slow the spread of the delta variant. Available at: https://www.whitehouse.gov/briefing-room/statements-releases/2021/07/29/fact-sheet-president-biden-to-announce-new-actions-to-get-more-americans-vaccinated-and-slow-the-spread-of-the-delta-variant. Accessed August 25, 2022.

Judicial Review of Public Health Powers Since the Start of the COVID-19 Pandemic: Trends and Implications

Wendy E. Parmet, JD, and Faith Khalik, JD

See also Parmet and Erwin, p. 267, Wiley, p. 269, Gostin, p. 272, Hodge et al., p. 275, and Platt et al., p. 288.

During the COVID-19 pandemic, officials in the United States at all levels of government utilized their legal authorities to impose a wide range of measures designed to control the spread of SARS-CoV-2 (severe acute respiratory syndrome coronavirus 2; the causative agent of COVID-19), including shutting down businesses, limiting the size of gatherings, requiring masking, and mandating vaccination.

These orders and regulations were challenged in court cases that resulted in more than 1000 judicial decisions. Common claims were based on alleged procedural and substantive due process violations, violations of religious liberty, and violations of officials' scope of authority. In more than three fourths of the decisions, the court refused to grant the plaintiffs the relief sought. However, plaintiffs found success in several notable cases, especially in federal court.

These recent decisions, as well as broader prepandemic trends, have important implications for public health officials' exercise of their public health powers, especially when those exercises implicate religious liberty. In this legal environment, officials may need to rely more on the powers of persuasion than on their legal authority alone. (*Am J Public Health*. 2023;113(3):280–287. https://doi.org/10.2105/AJPH.2022.307181)

AJPH March 2023, Vol 113, No. 3

Since March 2020, officials at all levels of government (federal, state, and local) have utilized their legal authorities to issue a wide range of orders and regulations designed to slow the transmission of SARS-CoV-2 (severe acute respiratory syndrome coronavirus 2; the causative agent of COVID-19). In response, individuals and entities around the country filed legal challenges. Courts have issued more than 1000 decisions in these cases.[1]

In more than three fourths of the more than 1000 decisions that we have collected, the court refused to give the plaintiff the relief sought. Nevertheless, some courts, including the US Supreme Court, have granted health officials less deference than they have traditionally received, especially in cases involving religious liberty or scope of authority.[2] This presents significant challenges to officials' ability to prevent and respond to future health threats. In the discussion that follows, we offer an overview of the decisions we have compiled, describe the courts' approaches to these claims, and consider the implications of these decisions for public health practice.

JUDICIAL DECISIONS DURING THE COVID-19 PANDEMIC

Using legal research methods, our team collected state and federal judicial decisions in Westlaw's legal database issued between March 1, 2020, and July 1, 2022, that relate to COVID-19 orders. Each decision in a case was counted separately. For example, we counted a trial court decision and a later appellate decision as 2 decisions. For the Supreme Court, we did not count denials of petition for *certiorari* but did include decisions on petitions for emergency relief (i.e., decisions from the so-called shadow docket) in which a justice or the majority wrote an opinion, including a concurrence or dissent. We did not include decisions that only discussed certain procedural or evidentiary matters, such as discovery motions. We also did not track tribal cases.

Search terms included topics such as "mask mandate," "face coverings,"

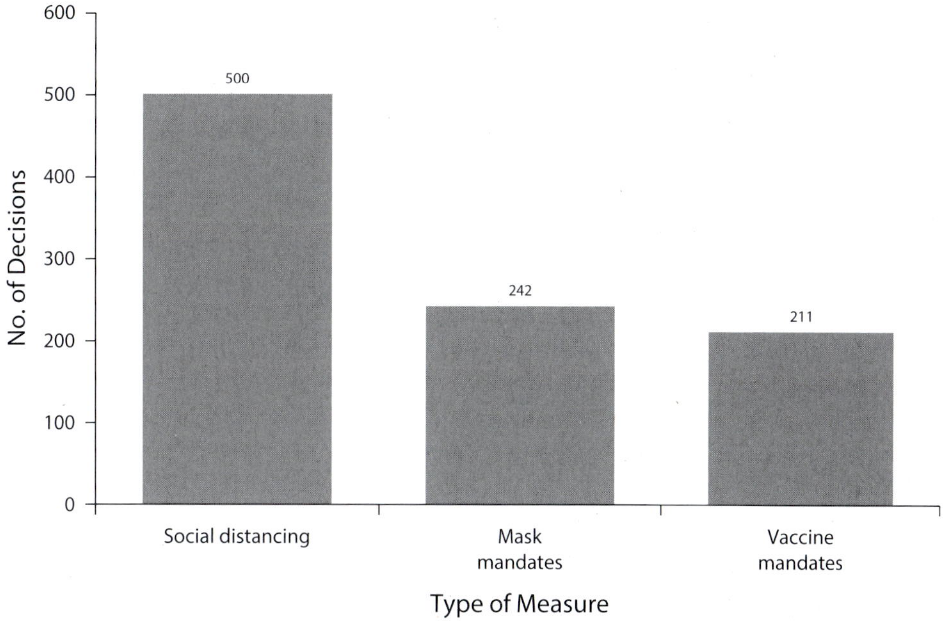

FIGURE 1— **Types of COVID-19 Response Measures Most Commonly Challenged: United States, March 2020–July 2022**

"quarantine," "vaccination requirements," "public health order," and "eviction moratorium," and legal issues such as "free exercise," "due process," "equal protection," "second amendment," and "administrative procedure."

We supplemented the decisions we found through Westlaw with decisions compiled by the Solomon Center for Health Law and Policy at Yale Law School, which also tracked COVID-19–related decisions. For each decision we found through either Westlaw or the Solomon Center's list, we utilized the "Citing References" function in Westlaw to find additional decisions. Each decision was entered into a spreadsheet and tagged by date, jurisdiction, topic, legal issues, and outcome. Each decision and its tags were subsequently reviewed by another research assistant or our senior researcher. Limitations to our approach include that we included decisions that were subsequently overruled or vacated, or, in the case of the Supreme Court, were signed by a minority of justices. We also did not give greater weight to precedential decisions. Nevertheless, our compilation sheds light on the landscape of judicial decisions concerning public health authorities during the pandemic.

The decisions that we collected dealt with the authority of government actors, including governors, state and federal agencies, city officials, health departments, and school districts. We did not include decisions that related solely to breach of contract claims, election procedures, immigration detention, or incarceration. We found 887 decisions in federal courts and 182 decisions in state courts. Most of the decisions dealt with challenges to state measures (945 decisions) versus federal measures (124 decisions). The measures most commonly discussed were social distancing measures (including business closures and restrictions, stay-at-home orders, and gathering restrictions; 500 decisions), mask mandates (242 decisions), and vaccine mandates (211 decisions; Figure 1). Many decisions discussed more than 1 of these issues.[1]

Not surprisingly, the mix of decisions followed the changing nature of the public health response to the pandemic. In 2020, most decisions dealt with business closures, stay-at-home orders, restrictions on gatherings (including for worship), and, later in the year, mask mandates. As restrictions on businesses and gatherings eased in 2021,[3] most decisions reviewed mask or vaccine mandates.

This article describes in further detail decisions analyzing legal claims relating to (1) individual rights, (2) scope of authority, and (3) administrative procedures.

INDIVIDUAL RIGHTS

Many of the public health orders issued during the pandemic restricted individual liberty and implicated (or at least potentially implicated) fundamental constitutional rights.[4] For example, stay-at-home orders affected the right to travel. Restrictions on worship raised issues relating to the First Amendment's guarantee of free exercise of religion.

Plaintiffs brought a wide range of individual rights claims. In 430 of the decisions we collected, plaintiffs argued that public health orders violated their rights under the Fourteenth Amendment to procedural due process, which concerns the process that is owed to an individual subjected to a government order, or substantive due process, which encompasses the right to privacy, including the right to abortion (before *Roe v Wade* was overturned). Courts ruled for plaintiffs in full or in part in 61 of these decisions.[1]

Equal protection claims were raised in 329 decisions we collected. Courts ruled for plaintiffs in full or in part in 45 of these decisions. Many plaintiffs argued that orders that shuttered or restricted some but not all businesses violated the Fourteenth Amendment's guarantee of equal protection. We collected 126 such decisions. For example, in *Big Tyme Investments v Edwards*, bar owners argued that Louisiana violated their right to equal protection by prohibiting the sale of alcohol and food at bars while allowing it in restaurants.[5] The US Court of Appeals for the Fifth Circuit disagreed, reasoning that because bars (unlike race or gender) is not a "suspect classification" for equal protection purposes, the plaintiffs had to prove that the government's order lacked a rational basis. The court then found that the plaintiff had not made such a showing. Most courts used similar reasoning to reject equal protection claims; in only 15 of the decisions we collected did courts rule partially or fully in favor of plaintiffs who raised such claims.

Several businesses alleged that COVID-19 orders, including eviction moratoria and shutdown orders, violated the Constitution's ban on impairment of contracts or its prohibition on the taking of property without just compensation. Courts ruled partially or fully in favor of plaintiffs in 16 of 149 decisions we found. For example, in *Auracle Homes v Lamont*, landlords argued that Connecticut's eviction moratorium "violates [their] constitutional rights under both the Contracts Clause and the Takings Clause of the US Constitution."[6] Denying plaintiffs a temporary restraining order, the US District Court in Connecticut reasoned that the Contracts Clause claim failed because the moratorium was reasonable and served a "significant and legitimate public purpose." The court rejected plaintiffs' takings claim because "reasonable investment-backed expectations cannot operate apart from 'public programs adjusting the benefits and burdens of economic life to promote the common good.'" Other decisions echoed this reasoning.

In 27 decisions, plaintiffs claimed that the state restricted their Second Amendment rights by closing gun stores or shooting ranges.[1] In 4 decisions, the court ruled that the order likely violated the Second Amendment. For example, in *Connecticut Citizens Defense League v Lamont*, the US District Court in Connecticut granted a preliminary injunction against Governor Lamont's executive order allowing police departments to suspend fingerprinting for obtaining a handgun permit, noting that "the courts retain a role to examine the use of governmental power even during a public health emergency."[7]

In spring 2020, 35 states had capacity limits or bans on gatherings that applied to in-person worship.[8] In at least 143 decisions, plaintiffs argued that these gathering restrictions violated the Free Exercise Clause of the First Amendment as well as, in some cases, statutory protections for religious liberty. Although most decisions rejected such claims, plaintiffs were more successful in these claims than in many other types of individual rights claims, as courts ruled partially or fully for plaintiffs in 37 of the 143 decisions in our compilation in which plaintiffs challenged gathering restrictions based on religious liberty claims.

In November 2020, the Supreme Court enjoined a New York order limiting the number of people who could gather for worship in COVID "hot zones," finding that it likely violated the Free Exercise Clause.[9] According to the court, the order was not neutral as to religion, and was therefore subject to strict scrutiny, the most stringent form of review. The court then ruled that the order failed strict scrutiny because it was not, in the court's assessment, the least restrictive means of achieving a compelling state interest. Over the next 6 months, the Supreme Court issued several additional decisions in favor of plaintiffs who challenged public health orders on free exercise grounds. In 3 of these decisions, the order that was challenged did not specify or explicitly target religion (Table 1). Nevertheless, most free exercise challenges continued to fail in the lower courts.

After restrictions on gatherings were lifted, religious liberty litigation focused on vaccine mandates. Plaintiffs argued that mandates without religious exemptions discriminated against religion by allowing medical, but not religious, exemptions.[10] Plaintiffs also challenged denials of religious exemptions that were available but were not granted to

TABLE 1— Supreme Court Opinions on Public Health Authorities Related to the COVID-19 Pandemic: United States

Case	Date	Disposition
Free Exercise Challenges to Restrictions on Gatherings		
South Bay United Pentecostal Church v Newsom (South Bay I), 140 S Ct 1613 (2020)	May 29, 2020	Plaintiffs' application for injunctive relief denied
Calvary Chapel Dayton Valley v Sisolak, 140 S Ct 2603 (2020)	Jul 24, 2020	Plaintiffs' application for injunctive relief denied
Roman Catholic Diocese of Brooklyn v Cuomo, 141 S Ct 63 (2020) (per curiam)	Nov 25, 2020	Plaintiffs' application for injunctive relief granted in part
Agudath Israel of America v Cuomo, 141 S Ct 889 (2020)	Nov 25, 2020	Plaintiffs' application for injunctive relief granted in part
Gateway City Church v Newsom, 141 S Ct 1460 (2021)	Dec 3, 2020	Plaintiffs' application for injunctive relief granted pending appeal and disposition of the petition for writ of certiorari
High Plains Harvest Church v Polis, 141 S Ct 527 (2020)	Dec 15, 2020	Plaintiffs' application for injunctive relief granted
Danville Christian Academy v Beshear, 141 S Ct 527 (2020)	Dec 17, 2020	Plaintiffs' application for a preliminary injunction denied
South Bay United Pentecostal Church v Newsom (South Bay II), 141 S Ct 716 (2021)	Feb 5, 2021	Plaintiffs' application for injunctive relief granted in part
Harvest Rock Church v Newsom, 141 S Ct 1289 (2021)	Feb 5, 2021	Plaintiffs' application for injunctive relief granted in part
Tandon v Newsom, 141 S Ct 1294 (2021) (per curiam)	Apr 9, 2021	Plaintiffs' application for injunctive relief granted
Free Exercise Challenges to Vaccine Mandates		
Does 1–3 v Mills, 142 S Ct 17 (2021)	Oct 29, 2021	Plaintiffs' application for injunctive relief denied
Dr A v Hochul, 142 S Ct 552 (2021)	Dec 13, 2021	Plaintiffs' application for injunctive relief denied
Austin v US Navy Seals 1–26, 142 S Ct 1301 (2022)	Mar 25, 2022	Government's application for a partial stay of the District Court's preliminary injunction granted
Scope of Authority Challenges		
Alabama Association of Realtors v HHS, 141 S Ct 2320 (2021)	Jun 29, 2021	Plaintiffs' application to vacate the lower court's stay of the CDC's national eviction moratorium denied
Chrysafis v Marks, 141 S Ct 2482 (2021)	Aug 12, 2021	Plaintiffs' application for injunctive relief granted
Alabama Association of Realtors v HHS, 141 S Ct 2485 (2021) (per curiam)	Aug 26, 2021	Plaintiffs' application to stay the CDC's nationwide eviction moratorium for residential rental properties granted
Biden v Missouri, 142 S Ct 647 (2022) (per curiam)	Jan 13, 2022	Government's application to stay preliminary injunctions granted
National Federation of Independent Businesses v OSHA, 142 S Ct 661 (2022) (per curiam)	Jan 13, 2022	Plaintiffs' application for a stay of OSHA's employee vaccination mandate granted

Note. CDC = Centers for Disease Control and Prevention; HHS = Department of Health and Human Services; OSHA = Occupational Safety and Health Administration. Only includes US Supreme Court cases between May 1, 2020, and July 1, 2022, in which there were opinions, including concurrences or dissents.

them as individuals. Although courts were more likely than not to rule against plaintiffs, plaintiffs were more successful with these cases than in many other individual rights claims, succeeding or partially succeeding in 21 of 81 free exercise vaccination decisions.

SCOPE OF AUTHORITY

For the most part, executive branch officials can only exercise powers granted to them by acts of the legislature through statutes. Each state has legislation granting the governor and other officials, at both the state and local levels, broad authority to respond to emergencies. Few of these statutes explicitly enumerate many of the measures used in response to COVID-19, such as stay-at-home orders or mask mandates. As a result, officials generally relied on broad statutory language that authorizes them to take actions that they find to be necessary to safeguard health or respond to an emergency.[11]

Many challengers argued that officials overstepped their authority by imposing measures that were not explicitly authorized by statute. Twenty cases challenging the scope of authority of state officials resulted in decisions by the state's supreme court, the final judicial authority on state statutory authority (Table 2). In 10 states, the high court affirmed officials' use of public health or emergency powers. For example, in *Grisham v Romero*, the New Mexico Supreme Court sided with

TABLE 2— State Supreme Court Decisions on Scope of Public Health Powers: United States, March 2020–July 2022

State	Upheld Exercise of Authority	Rejected or Blocked Exercise of Authority
Connecticut	*Casey v Lamont*, 258 A3d 647 (Conn 2021)	. . .
Florida	*Abramson v DeSantis*, 2020 WL 3464376 (Fla June 25, 2020)	. . .
Kansas	*Kelly v Legis Coordinating Council*, 460 P3d 832 (Kan 2020)	. . .
Kentucky	*Beshear v Acree*, 615 SW3d 780 (Ky 2020)	. . .
Massachusetts	*Desrosiers v Governor*, 158 NE3d 827 (Mass 2020)	. . .
Michigan	. . .	*House of Representatives v Governor*, 949 NW2d 276 (Mich 2020); *In re Certified Questions*, 506 Mich 332 (Mich 2020)
New Mexico	*Grisham v Romero*, 483 P3d 545 (NM 2021); *Grisham v Reeb*, 480 P3d 852 (NM 2020); *State v Wilson*, 489 P3d 925 (NM 2021)	. . .
North Dakota	*State v Riggin*, 959 NW2d 855 (ND 2021)	. . .
Oregon	*Elkhorn Baptist Church v Brown*, 466 P3d 30 (Or 2020)	. . .
Pennsylvania	*Friends of Danny DeVito v Wolf*, 227 A3d 872 (Pa 2020); *Wolf v Scarnati*, 233 A3d 679 (Pa 2020)	*Corman v Acting Secretary of Pennsylvania Department of Health*, 266 A3d 452 (Pa 2021)
Washington	*Matter of Recall of Inslee*, 508 P3d 635 (Wash 2022)	. . .
Wisconsin	. . .	*Tavern League of Wisconsin Inc v Palm*, 957 NW2d 261 (Wis 2021); *Fabick v Evers*, 956 NW2d 856 (Wis 2021); *Wisconsin Legis v Palm*, 942 NW2d 900 (Wis 2020); *James v Heinrich*, 960 NW2d 350 (Wis 2021)

Governor Lujan Grisham, stating that the Public Health Emergency Response Act granted her broad authority to impose measures to protect public health.[12] However, in 3 "purple" states with a Democratic governor and a Republican-led state legislature (Wisconsin, Michigan, and Pennsylvania), the state supreme court held that executive officials had exceeded the scope of their statutory authority. For example, in *Wisconsin v Palm*, the Republican-led state legislature argued that the Democratic governor's secretary-designee of the Department of Health Services exceeded her authority in issuing a stay-at-home order. The Wisconsin Supreme Court agreed.[13]

Four state supreme courts, all in states with divided government, also weighed in on governors' authority to declare or extend states of emergency (Table 2). Two courts (Kentucky and Massachusetts) held that the governors properly declared or extended a state of emergency. Two courts (Michigan and Wisconsin) held that the governors exceeded their authority by extending emergencies.

After the Biden administration took office, numerous scope of authority challenges were brought against federal orders, including the eviction moratorium issued by the Centers for Disease Control and Prevention (CDC), federal vaccine mandates, and mask mandates for travel. In August 2021, the Supreme Court relied on the relatively novel "major questions doctrine," which holds that administrative agencies cannot issue orders or regulations with major economic or political significance without explicit statutory authority, to block the CDC's eviction moratorium (Table 1). In January 2022, the court used that same doctrine to block an emergency rule by the Occupational Safety and Health Administration that would have required large employers to mandate either vaccination or testing and masking. The Supreme Court did permit the Centers for Medicare and Medicaid Services to require that health care workers be vaccinated, ruling that the agency had ample statutory authority to condition providers' participation in Medicare and Medicaid (Table 1). Following these decisions, lower federal courts have applied the major questions doctrine to block several other federal initiatives, including vaccine mandates for federal contractors[14] and the CDC's mask mandate for transportation.[15]

CHALLENGES BASED ON ADMINISTRATIVE PROCEDURES

State and federal administrative procedure acts require agencies, such as the CDC or state health departments, to go through a notice-and-comment process before enacting a rule. However, these acts usually allow agencies to bypass this process when it would be impractical, as in emergencies. Many plaintiffs challenged such emergency orders, arguing that agencies should have gone through the lengthier rule-making process.

Challenges on federal or state administrative procedure act grounds were more likely to be decided in favor of plaintiffs than challenges based on any other legal issue we tracked. Of the 85 relevant decisions we found, 33 ruled partially or fully in favor of plaintiffs.[1]

AN EVOLVING APPROACH TO JUDICIAL REVIEW

The exercise of public health powers can facilitate a quick and effective response to public health threats. Although far more research is needed, some studies have found that the use of such powers during the COVID-19 pandemic helped to reduce its toll.[16,17] Public health orders, however, can also be abused, as when San Francisco, California, targeted people of Asian descent during a bubonic plague outbreak in 1900.[18] Litigation and the judicial review it invokes can play a powerful role in preventing such abuses, ensuring that public health powers are utilized in a manner that is consistent with constitutional rights and the rule of law.

Traditionally, courts have granted health officials significant (but not total) deference when reviewing challenges to public health powers.[19] Most famously, in 1905 in *Jacobson v Massachusetts*, the Supreme Court expressed the importance of public health expertise when it upheld a vaccine mandate, explaining that the legislature could delegate the determination of whether a mandate was appropriate "to a board of health composed of persons residing in the locality affected, and appointed, presumably, because of their fitness to determine such questions."[20] The court concluded that the judiciary's role in reviewing such expert decisions should be limited.[20]

Even before the pandemic, judicial deference to public health powers was fading in response to challenges from both ends of the political spectrum.[21] Some legal scholars argued that courts should review public health orders more vigorously to safeguard constitutional liberties and reduce the misapplication of public health powers against minorities and vulnerable individuals.[22,23] Corporations and libertarians challenged public health laws relating to noncommunicable diseases as unduly paternalistic.[24] Some courts seemed convinced by such arguments. In 1 notable case, the New York Court of Appeals ruled that New York City's health department could not use its broad public health powers to limit portion sizes for sugary beverages.[25] Increased scrutiny of commercial speech regulations also led courts to block laws compelling graphic warnings for cigarettes and warnings in beverage advertisements.[21]

Despite these forewarnings, early in the COVID-19 pandemic, most courts noted the existence of a public health emergency and granted considerable (though varied) levels of deference to officials even when constitutionally protected rights were implicated.[26] In 1 widely cited case, the US Court of Appeals for the Fifth Circuit rejected a challenge to Texas Governor Greg Abbott's emergency order banning abortions, which at the time were still constitutionally protected, stating that during a public health emergency judicial review must be limited to determining if the order "has no real or substantial relation to [public health], or is, beyond all question, a plain, palpable invasion of rights."[27] A few weeks later, the Supreme Court in *South Bay United Pentecostal Church v Newsom* refused to block a California order restricting worship. Although the full court did not issue an opinion in that case, Chief Justice John Roberts wrote a concurring decision, stating, "Our Constitution principally entrusts 'the safety and the health of the people' to the politically accountable officials of the States."[28]

As the pandemic progressed and became more politically polarized, and especially after Justice Amy Coney Barrett replaced Ruth Bader Ginsburg on the high court, the Supreme Court appeared to grant officials less deference, especially in free exercise cases. This was initially evident in the court's decision to block New York's capacity limits on worship in hot zones.[9] Tellingly, the court in that case did not discuss *Jacobson*. Nor did it do so several months later when it ruled that a California order restricting gatherings of all types in private homes was subject to strict judicial scrutiny because it interfered with plaintiffs' ability to hold a Bible study group while some secular activities, like shopping, faced looser restrictions.[29] In reaching that conclusion, and in contrast with Chief Justice Roberts' call for deference in *South Bay*, the majority gave no weight to health officials' determination that gatherings in private homes were different from and more dangerous than the public gatherings that were less strictly regulated. Indeed, the court did not discuss any of the public health evidence in the record.

The Supreme Court's new stance toward free exercise claims opened the door to religious liberty challenges to vaccine mandates. Before the pandemic, courts uniformly rejected such claims.[10] Since 2021, the courts have been divided as to whether public vaccine mandates must include religious exemptions, or whether the denial of a requested exemption is unconstitutional. For example, in *US Navy Seals 1–26 v Biden*, the Fifth Circuit ruled that the Navy's failure to grant religious exemptions likely violated service members' statutory rights to religious liberty. In reaching that conclusion, the court rejected the Navy's contention that its vaccine mandate was essential to ensuring the safety and readiness of the troops.[30] The Supreme Court narrowed the injunction in that case, allowing the Navy to consider "respondents' vaccination status in deployment, assignment, and other operational decisions" but still preventing the Navy from enforcing the vaccination requirement on plaintiffs.[31] Conversely, federal appellate courts in the First and Second Circuits rejected religious challenges to vaccine mandates for health care workers.[32,33] To date, the Supreme Court has chosen not to consider a free exercise challenge to a state vaccine mandate. Several justices, however, published opinions arguing that states' failure to provide religious exemptions violates the Constitution.[34] These statements, when combined with the Supreme Court's new approach to religious liberty claims, may invite challenges to childhood vaccine laws and many other public health measures that individuals may believe interfere with their religious practices or views.[10]

Using the major questions doctrine and related approaches to statutory construction, the Supreme Court and some lower courts have also begun to read broad delegations of public health powers narrowly to prohibit officials from issuing measures that are not explicitly enumerated in a statute. This cramped reading of public health statutes can make it difficult for health officials to respond to novel health problems that require interventions that legislatures could not have anticipated. It also means that officials must wait for the legislature to act before issuing needed orders or risk having them struck down. Political gridlock and the fact that most state legislatures do not meet year-round compound the problem.

IMPLICATIONS FOR PUBLIC HEALTH PRACTICE

Although courts continue to reject most challenges to public health measures, decisions issued during the COVID-19 pandemic show that health officials cannot assume that courts will give them the benefit of the doubt. In this climate, it is more essential than ever that health officials base their decisions on the best available science and assemble a robust record that can demonstrate the necessity of their actions. This may not forestall litigation or guarantee success in it, but it is an essential first step.

Officials also need to take special care when issuing orders that may touch upon religious practices and beliefs. Public health measures that specify religious practices, such as limitations on worship, face heighted constitutional risk, but so do orders that are neutral on their face as to religion but may still interfere with an individual's ability to practice their faith. In particular, laws that appear to restrict an exercise of religion more strictly than "comparable" secular activities (even if the scientific evidence does not back up that comparability) may be subject to strict judicial scrutiny and held unconstitutional. To avoid this risk, officials should ensure that the lines they draw are grounded in the best available science. Officials must also understand that simply providing religious exemptions on paper will not insulate a mandate or other order from a free exercise challenge; they must have strong evidence to justify denying any religious exemptions that are requested. Even then, the order may be struck.

Given the high percentage of administrative procedure cases won by plaintiffs, officials should consider commencing rule-making procedures as quickly as possible if they want emergency orders to stay in place. When a new health threat, such as a pandemic, strikes, officials need to act swiftly; rule-making is often impossible at that point. But as a pandemic or other emergency continues, the rule-making process can avoid some legal problems and enable the public to weigh in on whether particular health measures should continue.

Most importantly, health officials need to recognize both the extent and limits of their legal powers. Officials continue to win most cases and should not be dissuaded from issuing critical orders or regulations because of overblown fears of litigation. The decisions issued during the COVID-19 pandemic show that, especially in the early days of a health threat, most courts will still give officials considerable deference.

Nevertheless, public health officials have lost some very important, high-profile cases. In addition, the very process of litigation, even when the outcome is successful from a public health perspective, can deplete resources and distract officials from doing their job. Further, in our highly polarized political climate, officials need to accept that litigation can play a politically performative role, in which partisans run to court to challenge and politically weaken their opponents, as when the Republican legislature challenged the Democratic governor's public health orders in Wisconsin[13] or when several "red states" challenged Biden's vaccine mandates.[1]

In this legal environment, health officials should remember that persuasion is among their most potent powers. A public that distrusts or doesn't understand health measures is more likely to challenge them in court. And judges may find it easier to strike orders that are deeply unpopular. Conversely, a public that trusts public health authorities and understands the rationale for recommended measures is probably less likely to litigate. Although obtaining the public's support can be difficult in the current political and informational climate, it will be increasingly essential if the judiciary further constricts officials' legal authorities. Although many health departments face limited resources, investing in training or additional help in communicating with the public may be well worth the costs, leading to better outcomes and decreased litigation. AJPH

ABOUT THE AUTHORS

Wendy E. Parmet and Faith Khalik are with the Center for Health Policy & Law, Northeastern University School of Law, Boston, MA.

CORRESPONDENCE

Correspondence should be sent to Wendy E. Parmet, Center for Health Policy & Law, Northeastern University School of Law, 416 Huntington Ave, Boston, MA 02115 (e-mail: w.parmet@northeastern.edu). Reprints can be ordered at http://www.ajph.org by clicking the "Reprints" link.

PUBLICATION INFORMATION

Full Citation: Parmet WE, Khalik F. Judicial review of public health powers since the start of the COVID-19 pandemic: trends and implications. *Am J Public Health.* 2023;113(3):280–287.

Acceptance Date: November 16, 2022.

DOI: https://doi.org/10.2105/AJPH.2022.307181

CONTRIBUTORS

Each author contributed to conceptualizing and writing the article. F. Khalik oversaw the compilation of cases discussed in the article.

ACKNOWLEDGMENTS

Research was supported by a grant from the Robert Wood Johnson Foundation (via ChangeLab Solutions) as a component of the Act for Public Health Initiative.

Research assistance was provided by Julia Winett, Gavin Hunter, Robert Benjamin McMichael, Marcus Jones, John Matthew Catoe, Catherine Kuchel, Kyla Portnoy, and Julia Brown. Many thanks to Scott Burris for his comments on an earlier draft of this article.

CONFLICTS OF INTEREST

The authors have no conflicts of interest to disclose.

HUMAN PARTICIPANT PROTECTION

This study did not involve any human participants.

REFERENCES

1. Public Health Law Watch. List of Public Health Authority cases as of 7/1/2022. Available at: https://www.publichealthlawwatch.org/pha7122. Accessed November 10, 2022.
2. Mello MM, Parmet WE. US public health law—foundations and emerging shifts. *N Engl J Med.* 2022;386(9):805–808. https://doi.org/10.1056/NEJMp2200794
3. International Monetary Fund. Policy responses to COVID-19. Updated July 2, 2021. Available at: https://www.imf.org/en/Topics/imf-and-covid19/Policy-Responses-to-COVID-19. Accessed November 7, 2022.
4. Network for Public Health Law. Individual rights and the public's health: constitutional, ethical, and political aspects of COVID-19 measures and their enforcement. February 24, 2021. Available at: https://www.networkforphl.org/news-insights/individual-rights-and-the-publics-health-constitutional-ethical-and-political-aspects-of-covid-19-measures-and-their-enforcement. Accessed November 7, 2022.
5. *Big Tyme Investments LLC v Edwards*, 985 F3d 456 (5th Cir 2021).
6. *Auracle Homes LLC v Lamont*, 478 F Supp3d 199 (D Conn 2020).
7. *Connecticut Citizens Defense League v Lamont*, 465 F Supp3d 56 (D Conn 2020).
8. Villa V. Most states have religious exemptions to COVID-19 social distancing rules. Pew Research Center. April 27, 2020. Available at: https://www.pewresearch.org/fact-tank/2020/04/27/most-states-have-religious-exemptions-to-covid-19-social-distancing-rules. Accessed August 2, 2022.
9. *Roman Catholic Diocese of Brooklyn v Cuomo*, 141 S Ct 63 (2020) (per curiam).
10. Parmet WE. From the shadows: the public health implications of the Supreme Court's COVID-free exercise cases. *J Law Med Ethics.* 2021;49(4):564–579. https://doi.org/10.1017/jme.2021.80
11. Wiley LF. Democratizing the law of social distancing. *Yale J Health Policy Law Ethics.* 2020;19(3):50–121. https://doi.org/10.2139/ssrn.3634997
12. *Grisham v Romero*, 483 P3d 545 (NM 2021).
13. *Wisconsin Legislature v Palm*, 942 NW2d 900 (Wis 2020).
14. *Georgia v Biden*, 574 F Supp3d 1337 (SD Ga 2021).
15. *Health Freedom Defense Fund Inc v Biden*, 2022 WL 1134138 (MD Fla April 18, 2022).
16. Huang J, Fisher BT, Tam V, et al. The effectiveness of government masking mandates on COVID-19 county-level case incidence across the United States, 2020. *Health Aff (Millwood).* 2022;41(3):445–453. https://doi.org/10.1377/hlthaff.2021.01072
17. Zhang X, Warner ME. COVID-19 policy differences across US states: shutdowns, reopening, and mask mandates. *Int J Environ Res Public Health.* 2020;17(24):9520. https://doi.org/10.3390/ijerph17249520
18. *Jew Ho v Williamson*, 103 F 10 (ND Cal 1900).
19. Gostin LO. *Jacobson v Massachusetts* at 100 years: police power and civil liberties in tension. *Am J Public Health.* 2005;95(4):576–581. https://doi.org/10.2105/AJPH.2004.055152
20. *Jacobson v Massachusetts*, 197 US 11 (1905).
21. Parmet WE, Jacobson PD. The courts and public health: caught in a pincer movement. *Am J Public Health.* 2014;104(3):392–397. https://doi.org/10.2105/AJPH.2013.301738
22. Mariner WK, Annas GJ, Glantz LH. *Jacobson v Massachusetts*: it's not your great-great-grandfather's public health law. *Am J Public Health.* 2005;95(4):581–590. https://doi.org/10.2105/AJPH.2004.055160
23. Gostin LO, Burris S, Lazzarini Z. The law and the public's health: a study of infectious disease law in the United States. *Columbia Law Rev.* 1999;99(1):59–128. https://doi.org/10.2307/1123597
24. Sullivan S. Tobacco talk: why FDA tobacco advertising restrictions violate the First Amendment. *William Mitchell Law Rev.* 1997;23:743–785.
25. *NY Statewide Coalition of Hispanic Chambers of Commerce v New York City Dep't of Health & Mental Hygiene*, 16 NE3d 538 (NY 2014).
26. Mok K, Posner EA. Constitutional challenges to public health orders in federal courts during the COVID-19 pandemic. *BU Law Review.* 2022;102:1729–1785.
27. *In re Abbott*, 954 F3d 772, 784 (quoting *Jacobson v Massachusetts*, 197 US at 31).
28. *South Bay United Pentecostal Church v Newsom*, 140 S Ct 1613 (2020) (Roberts, CJ, concurring).
29. *Tandon v Newsom*, 141 S Ct 1294 (2021) (per curiam).
30. *US Navy Seals 1–26 v Biden*, 27 F4th 336 (5th Cir 2022).
31. *Austin v US Navy Seals 1–26*, 142 S Ct 1301 (2022).
32. *Does 1–6 v Mills*, 16 F4th 20 (1st Cir 2021).
33. *We The Patriots USA v Hochul*, 17 F4th 266 (2d Cir 2021).
34. *Dr A v Hochul*, 142 S Ct 552 (2021) (Gorsuch, J, dissenting).

Trends in US State Public Health Emergency Laws, 2021–2022

Elizabeth Platt, JD, MA, Katie Moran-McCabe, JD, Amy Cook, JD, and Scott Burris, JD

See also Parmet and Erwin, p. 267, Wiley, p. 269, Gostin, p. 272, Hodge et al., p. 275, and Parmet and Khalik, p. 280.

Objectives. To identify and categorize US state legislation introduced between January 1, 2021, and May 20, 2022, that addresses emergency health authority.

Methods. We adapted standard policy surveillance methods to collect and code state bills and enacted laws limiting or expanding the emergency public health authority of state and local officials and agencies.

Results. State legislators introduced 1531 bills addressing public health authority; 191 of those were enacted in 43 states and the District of Columbia, including 17 expanding and 65 contracting emergency authority, 163 regulating use, and 30 preempting local use of specific measures such as mask mandates.

Conclusions. State laws setting the scope and limits of emergency authority are crucial to effective public health response. These laws are changing in ways that threaten to reduce response capacity. Tracking changes in health law infrastructure is important for evaluating changes in health authority and ensuring that stakeholders recognize these changes.

Public Health Implications. The COVID-19 pandemic called for quick, decisive action to limit infections, and when the next outbreak hits, new laws limiting health authority will make such action even more difficult. (*Am J Public Health*. 2023;113(3):288–296. https://doi.org/10.2105/AJPH.2022.307214)

AJPH March 2023, Vol 113, No. 3

In the US legal system, states have the primary responsibility for enacting pandemic control measures. State legislatures define the nature and extent of public health agency authority and the emergency powers of governors and mayors, which are crucial to public health preparedness and response. Executive agencies are the first responders to unexpected events, such as a new pathogen. Their capacity to obtain and interpret information and subsequently launch appropriate testing, vaccination, treatment, and nonpharmaceutical interventions provides the best chance of preventing a major outbreak. The ability of health officials to do this work depends in significant part on what the law requires or allows.

Flexible authority to manage epidemics and other emergencies was built into US public health law at least as far back as the first boards of health at the turn of the 19th century.[1] From the legal point of view, public health administration has depended on 2 distinct features of the law: (1) grants of authority to officials typically included a catchall reference to "any other actions" the health officer deemed necessary in response to unanticipated health threats, and (2) courts tended to interpret this residual authority broadly and with deference.[1,2] In modern times, mechanisms for declaring official emergencies and triggering broad powers were added to state (and federal) law. Thus, as COVID-19 struck, federal, state, and local officials were able to respond rapidly with sweeping emergency orders.[3]

Initially, courts upheld these measures, deferring to the judgments of health officials.[3] As COVID-19 control measures grew more tendentious in politics and public opinion, fewer judges deferred, and a shifting Supreme Court majority adopted new doctrines of general administrative law that limit health and other administrative agencies to powers and measures expressly stated in law and applied First and Second Amendment protections more stringently.[4] As courts examine health measures with less deference and interpret the law more narrowly, the ability of state and local officials to address health threats depends more than ever on the language of state health laws defining their powers.

This body of state public health law is changing. In the legislative sessions starting in January 2021, state legislators introduced more than 1500 bills to change the legal authority of state and local health agencies and executive officers. In our legal mapping research, we documented state bills that affected the nature or allocation of public health authority at the state and local levels and state laws limiting public health emergency authority from January 1, 2021, through May 20, 2022. Our results provide an initial look at the authority state and local officials will have—and the political headwinds they will face—as they manage major threats to public health in the future.

METHODS

We adapted standard policy surveillance methods[5] to support rapid collection and reporting of bill and enacted law data. Legal researchers defined the topical scope of the research and developed a coding scheme. A commercial bill-tracking firm engaged by the Association of State and Territorial Health Officials identified legislation covering January 1, 2021, to May 20, 2022, using proprietary methods. The Association of State and Territorial Health Officials screened identified bills and laws and transmitted them to the Center for Public Health Law Research collaborating team. Data, codebooks, and research protocols are available at lawatlas.org.

Bills Addressing Public Health Authority

We included bills if they set limits on authority to declare public health emergencies or issue emergency orders ("limits on health authority"), changed the agency or official responsible for an emergency public health response ("public health authority reallocation"), expanded the emergency authority of a public health agency or official ("public health authority expansions"), limited state or local enforcement of federal health mandates ("limits on federal laws"), regulated the deployment of specific response measures ("regulation of emergency measures"), or preempted local public health authority to enact emergency control measures ("preemption of emergency measures"). We organized each category of bills as a separate longitudinal data set.

We checked identified bills against a separate list compiled by collaborating attorneys from the Network for Public Health Law, who reviewed state legislative Web sites, news media reports, and personal communications to identify bills in the regions they serve. Six Center for Public Health Law Research attorneys individually assigned bills to topical data sets and coded the variables on the policy-tracking software MonQcle (Center for Public Health Law Research, Philadelphia, PA). We resolved ambiguous cases through further review and group discussion. We logged definitions and coding rules into research protocol notes shared among the team for cohesiveness. Supervising attorneys reviewed final coding.

Laws Limiting Public Health Authority

We created 1 longitudinal data set of enacted laws that limited public health authority. Researchers used search alerts from the Westlaw legal research platform and active keyword searches on openstates.org to verify initial research and identify missing laws. We used Westlaw to check for further amendments for each law in the data set. One researcher coded each record, and a supervising attorney reviewed the data set.

RESULTS

From the beginning of the 2021–2022 state legislative sessions to May 20, 2022, legislators introduced 1531 total bills to change the scope and allocation of emergency health authority generally or with respect to COVID-19 (Table 1). The most common type of bill regulated the use of specific control measures, such as vaccination, testing, and masks,

TABLE 1— Introduced and Enacted US State Legislation Addressing Public Health Authority by Topic: January 1, 2021–May 20, 2022

Topic	Introduced Bills, No.	Enacted Bills, % (No.)
Federal enforcement limits	27	18.5 (5)
Preemption	177	16.9 (30)
Authority expansion	102	16.7 (17)
Emergency measures regulation	1197	13.6 (163)
Authority limits	539	12.1 (65)
Authority reallocation	84	7.1 (6)
All bills	1531	12.5 (191)

Note: Because bills may address more than 1 topic, totals reported by topic will not sum to the total number of bills.

followed by bills that limited the public health authority of a governor, state health official, or local health official. Bills frequently addressed multiple topics, so totals reported by category will not sum to the total number of bills. Interactive maps and tables containing state-level details—including bill text—about the legislation for each topic can be found on lawatlas.org.

As of May 20, 2022, 191 of the 1531 bills were enacted into law in 43 states and the District of Columbia, including 7 via veto override. Of those, 554 failed (i.e., were voted down or expired at the end of the session), 7 remained vetoed, and 779 remained in consideration at the end of our observation period. States saw an average of 30 introduced bills, with a range of 3 (Delaware) to 113 (New York). States enacted an average of 4 laws, ranging from none in 7 states (DE, IL, MA, MI, MO, NM, and RI) to 13 in Virginia. In states that enacted a law, pass rates as a percentage of all bills introduced varied from 1% in Minnesota to 80% in North Dakota.

Laws Expanding Public Health Authority

Twelve states (CO, GA, IN, LA, MD, NJ, OR, PA, SC, VA, VT, and WV) passed 17 laws expanding emergency authority. Expansion measures included laws that enhanced the organizational independence of health agencies (Colorado House Bill 22-1352), expanded authority during the COVID-19 pandemic (Indiana House Bill 1001, Pennsylvania House Bill 1861), or created new emergency rule-making procedures (Louisiana Senate Bill 136). Three states both expanded and contracted emergency response options: Georgia authorized local health authorities to disseminate vaccination information to manage a disease outbreak (Georgia Senate Bill 46) but also barred state and local governments from requiring proof of COVID-19 vaccination (Georgia Senate Bill 345). Indiana authorized state health authorities to issue standing orders, prescriptions, or protocols for immunizations (Indiana House Bill 1001) but also prohibited the state from requiring a COVID-19 vaccine passport (Indiana House Bill 1405). New Jersey passed a law establishing a COVID-19 pandemic task force on health disparities (New Jersey Assembly Bill 4004), coded as an expansion, but also terminated the governor's COVID-19 public health emergency and several executive orders (New Jersey Assembly Bill 5820).

Laws Limiting Emergency Authority

Twenty-five states enacted 65 laws that limited the emergency authority of governors, other state officials, or local health officials (Figure 1; Table A, available as a supplement to the online version of this article at http://www.ajph.org). Figure 1 shows the types of limitations and the officials subject to them. Most common were laws limiting the scope of orders, with 21 states enacting 54 such laws. Idaho, for example, enacted 4 laws that limited emergency authority to measures "essential to protect life or property from the occurrence or imminent threat of the state of [*sic*] disaster emergency threatening the safety of persons or property" (Idaho House Bill 393) and prohibited the governor and all other state and local officials from limiting "any rights guaranteed by the United States constitution or constitution of the state of Idaho, including but not limited to the right to peaceable assembly or free exercise of religion" (Idaho House Bill 391); prohibited the governor from altering or creating any provision of the Idaho Code during a disaster emergency (Idaho House Bill 392); and required that emergency orders "be narrowly focused without placing unnecessary restrictions on the ability for a person . . . to work, provide for their families, or otherwise contribute to the economy" (Idaho Senate Bill 1217).

Sixteen states enacted 20 laws that limited the issuance of emergency orders, for example by requiring that an executive order be submitted to a Legislative Council for review. In Montana, the law now states that after declaring a state of emergency, the governor "may not declare another state of emergency or disaster based on the same or substantially similar facts and circumstances without legislative approval" (Montana House Bill 230).

Fifteen states enacted 18 laws limiting the duration of emergencies. Limits averaged 33 days, ranging from 90 in Ohio (Ohio Senate Bill 22) to as few as 10 in Wyoming (for a stay-at-home order to limit the transmission of a contagious disease; Wyoming House Bill 127).

Eleven states enacted 16 laws addressing termination of emergency orders by the legislature or another entity. For example, Florida Senate Bill 2006 added a provision that allowed the legislature to terminate emergency orders by concurrent resolution, whereas Montana House Bill 121 allowed local health official orders to be terminated by county commissioners or other local elected officials. Kansas enacted Senate Bill 40, which limited gubernatorial orders by allowing local governments to supersede them with less strict rules.

Laws Reallocating Emergency Authority

We categorized a law as "reallocating" authority when it removed an

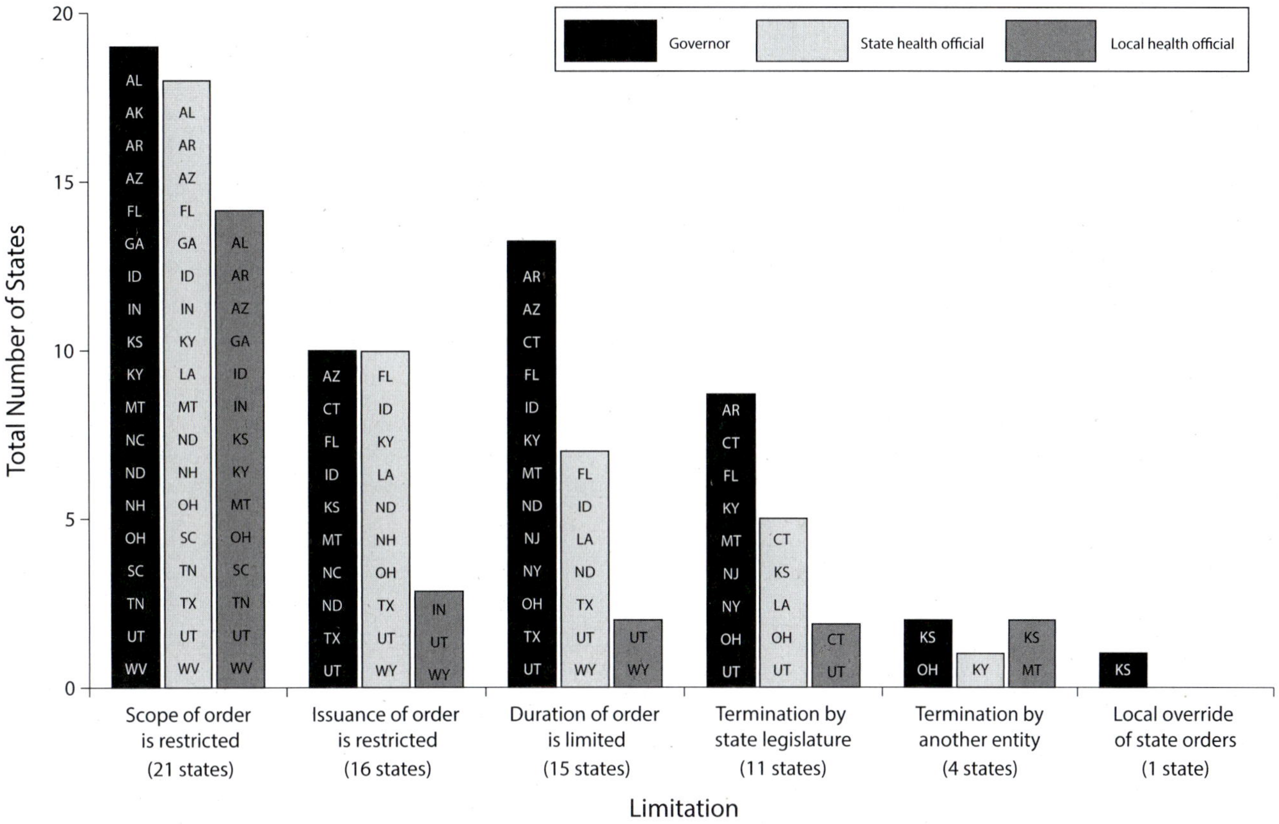

FIGURE 1— Types of Limitation of Public Health Emergency Authority and Officials Subject to Them in US State Legislation: January 1, 2021–May 20, 2022

emergency power from a governor or health official and gave it to the legislature or another official or agency. Six laws in 6 states reallocated authority. For example, Kansas Senate Bill 40 requires that county commissioners approve local health officer orders mandating the use of face masks, limiting gatherings, or restricting business operations.

Laws Limiting Federal Enforcement

Five states (ID, MT, SC, UT, and WY) enacted laws purporting to regulate the enforcement of federal public health laws or orders by state or local officials. In the US federal system, state officers are generally permitted, but not required, to enforce federal laws. These measures eliminate that discretion. For example, South Carolina House Bill 3126 provides that a federal vaccine mandate shall not be enforced unless a state or federal court holds it to be enforceable. Wyoming House Bill 1002 states that no public entity shall enforce any federal rule requiring an employer to mandate that employees receive a COVID-19 vaccination.

Laws Regulating Specific Measures Use

Forty-one states and the District of Columbia enacted 163 laws that addressed state executive or local authority to impose specific disease control measures, including mask mandates, vaccination requirements, and school or business closures (Figure 2). Some laws enhanced or otherwise supported authority to deploy these measures. For example, Virginia required the Department of Health to establish a volunteer program for eligible health care providers to administer the severe acute respiratory syndrome coronavirus 2 (SARS-CoV-2) vaccinations (Virginia House Bill 2333 and Senate Bill 1445), and New York made it a crime to falsify SARS-CoV-2 vaccination records (New York Assembly Bill 8700 and Senate Bill 4516). Other laws restricted authority. Iowa prohibited school districts from adopting or enforcing face mask requirements and prohibited the mandatory disclosure of vaccination status (Iowa House File 847 and House File 889). Some states enacted both kinds of laws. More than half of these laws (57%)—55 of 95 restrictive measures and 38 of 68 expansive measures—applied exclusively to COVID-19,

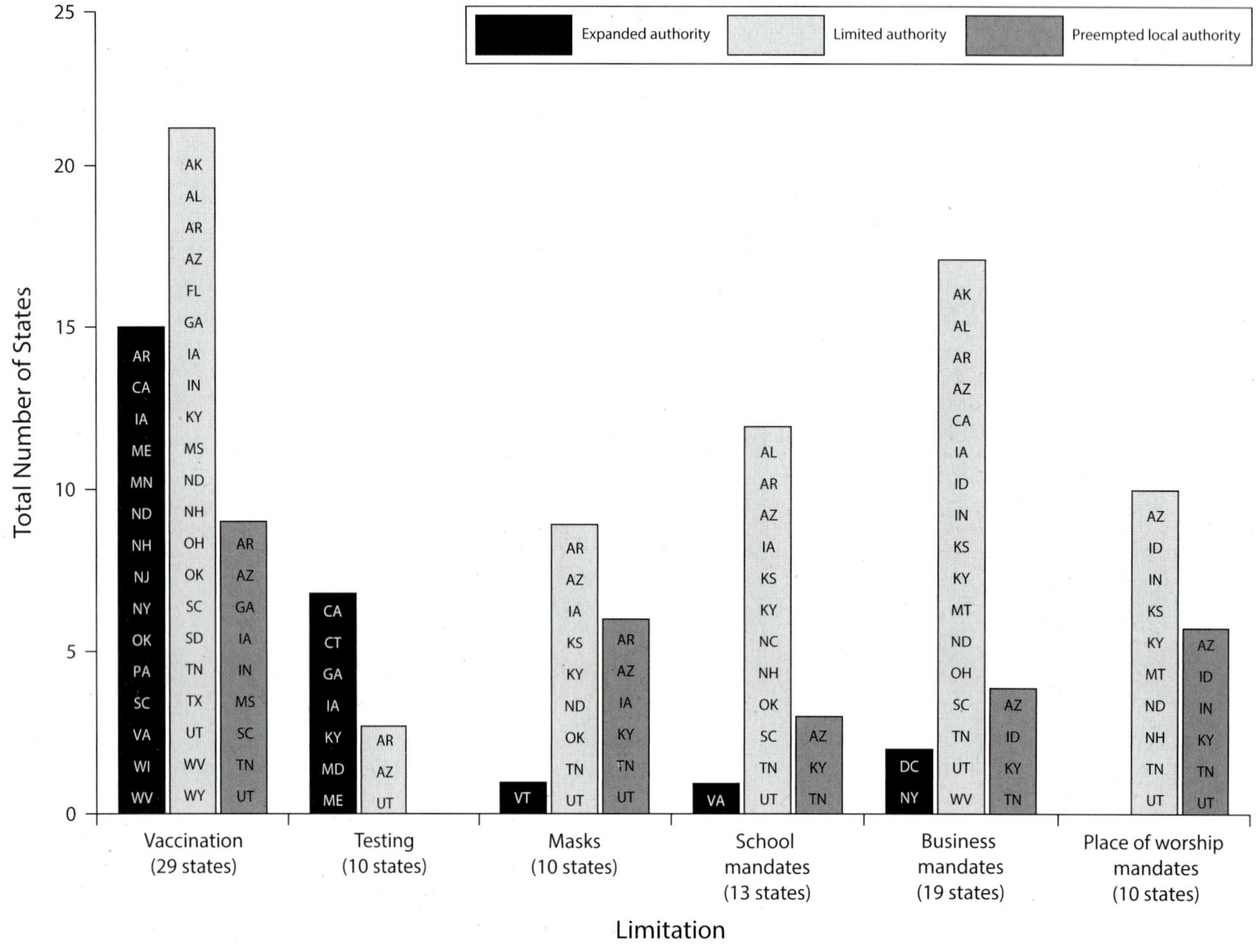

FIGURE 2— US States That Enacted Legislation Expanding, Restricting, or Locally Preempting Public Health Measures: January 1, 2021–May 20, 2022

so they will not apply to other threats now or in the future (Table B, available as a supplement to the online version of this article at http://www.ajph.org).

Twelve states enacted 30 laws that preempted local authorities from implementing 1 or more specific health measures. Vaccine requirements were the most common targets, followed by mask mandates and limits on religious gatherings. Almost half (14) of these apply exclusively to COVID-19 (Table B).

Party Control

There was little partisan difference in the intensity of legislative activity, but there was a striking difference in outcome. The 15 states that saw the most bill introductions were fairly evenly divided between Republican and Democratic control of the legislature and governorship, but all except 1 (CT) of the states that enacted more than 1 restrictive public health measure bill had Republican control of the legislature (Figure 3; Table C, available as a supplement to the online version of this article at http://www.ajph.org).

DISCUSSION

Public health law reform is to be expected after a major shock. The terrorist attacks and severe acute respiratory syndrome outbreak early in this century were both followed by significant attention to laws governing emergency preparedness and response.[6,7] Research demonstrates the high prevalence of emergency laws and the complexity of implementation networks they created.[8] Public health lawyers have analyzed responses to the emergencies and developed the Model State Emergency Health Powers Act,[6,9] which was subjected to robust public debate.[10,11] More than 40 states adopted 1 or more of its provisions over the following decade.[12] By contrast, legislation responding to COVID-19 has been highly politically partisan, rapid, and

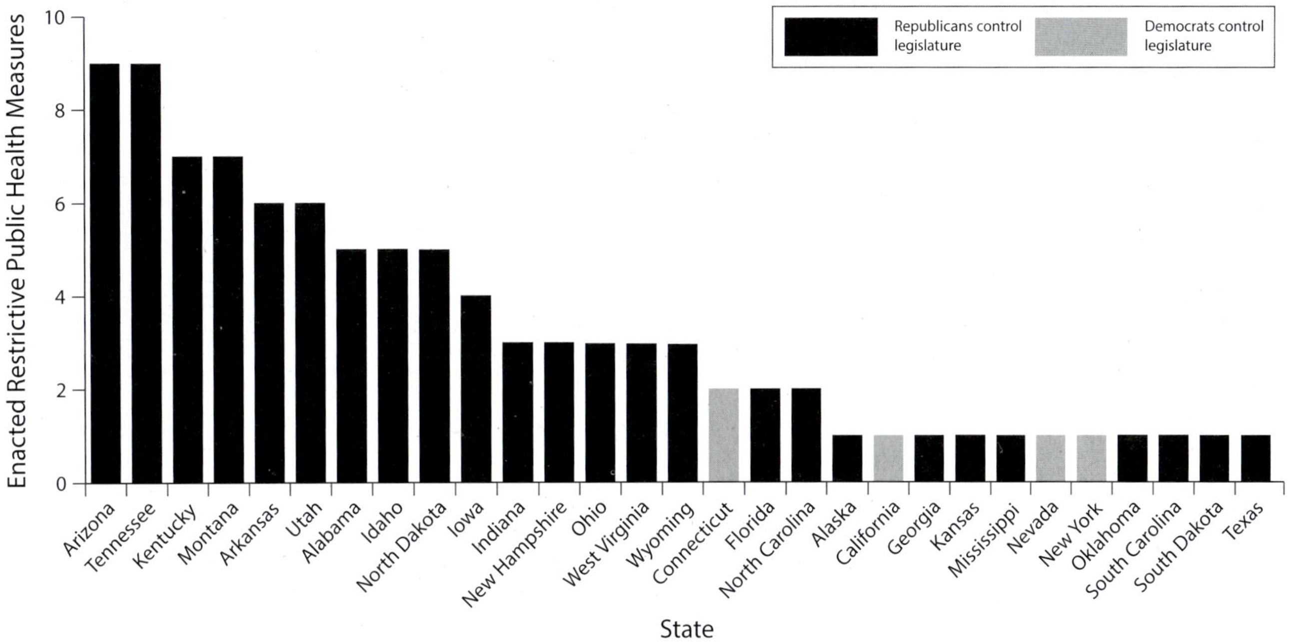

FIGURE 3— Enacted US State Legislation Restricting Public Health Measures by State and Party Control of Legislature: January 1, 2021–May 20, 2022

uninformed by careful and sustained research and analysis of the COVID-19 emergency response. In the first legislative session after COVID-19 hit, most states changed their law in some way.

The most frequently introduced and enacted laws addressed specific public health measures. These laws, more than half of which were specific to COVID-19, restrict measures that could reduce morbidity and mortality in the continuing COVID-19 pandemic; they reflect legislative interest in setting policy for COVID-19 without changing public health authority generally. Twenty-five states enacted laws limiting state or local officials' authority to respond to public health emergencies (Table A). Laws that limit the scope and duration of emergency orders or that shift emergency authority from executives to legislatures are concerning because they impose arbitrary limits on the discretion of the officials charged with taking action.

Although the duration of COVID-19 measures strained common expectations of how long an emergency should last, the experience also suggests that state legislatures, many of which were not even in session, are not institutionally disposed or well suited to enacting emergency legislation or managing response during a health crisis. Similarly, some new laws were written, unintentionally or intentionally, in ways that may chill the actual use of powers and invite court challenges. Idaho's new law, for example, will require health officials to be confident that emergency measures are essential to address an imminent threat and to be prepared for court challenges contending that the measures are not narrowly tailored enough. Laws like these pose a serious threat to the state's practical ability to respond in a timely way to an emergency.

Contextualizing legislative activity quantitatively is difficult because the output of legislatures is not systematically tracked. On average, state legislators reportedly introduce more than 109 000 bills each session.[13] On average, according to a commercial bill-tracking company, 20% of introduced bills are enacted, but state enactment rates vary from 5% to more than 60%.[14] An analysis of the 2012–2014 state legislative sessions, using data from the same tracking firm we used, found 804 bills across 12 health law domains, including housing and chronic disease control and core public health powers. Of these, only 13 addressed emergency preparedness and response. Of the 804 bills, 242 were enacted into law, including 5 of the 13 dealing with emergency preparedness.[15] These reports are consistent with the perception that the amount of public health emergency powers legislation was dramatically higher than usual in the 2021–2022 session.

Bills do not reflect actual levels of legislator or public interest in or concern about an issue. Any legislator can introduce a bill, allowing proposals that are best described as bizarre and that legislators do not give serious consideration. For example, New Hampshire House Bill 1027 sought to establish the crime of "undermining the legislative process by false claim of emergency" and accused President Biden of colluding with the Occupational Safety and Health Administration to bypass the legislative process under a false claim of an emergency. Several bills were introduced that allowed pharmacists and physicians to prescribe ivermectin and hydroxychloroquine for preventing COVID-19.

Historically, disputes over the division of authority in government are common. There is no correct division of power. Each entity has its strengths and weaknesses in terms of efficiency, accountability, and innovation. In practice, the allocation tends to be a matter of politics rather than rational, evidence-informed governance optimization.[16,17]

It is well established that in the United States, industry and conservative political forces have worked to limit the public health authority of liberal cities in relation to conservative state legislatures and to use state law to limit health regulation generally.[18–23] State legislatures' widespread preemption of local health and welfare legislation is a well-documented problem,[19,21] and research has suggested that preemption has harmful health effects.[24] In the case of public health powers, organized efforts include a model emergency powers law written by the American Legislative Exchange Council. The American Legislative Exchange Council Emergency Power Limitation Act would subject all emergency measures to the most stringent constitutional standard ("narrowly tailored to serve a compelling state interest") and set an automatic expiration date of as few as 7 days for executive orders.[25] Our research team identified at least 26 bills limiting public health authority as identical to or based on the American Legislative Exchange Council model. The fact that new limits on authority have been concentrated in "red" states is worrisome in light of evidence that conservative state legislatures' policy choices are already causing disparities in state life expectancy.[26]

Events in the courts have made the scope and language of state laws more important. Courts, including the Supreme Court, have increasingly adopted major questions and general nondelegation rules that require grants of authority to administrative agencies, including health departments, to be explicit and specific.[27] Construing state and federal law according to these doctrines parallels the much older practice of narrowly interpreting state grants of authority to local governments, an approach that has limited local health authority in many states.[28]

COVID-19 revealed problems with public health capacity and professional culture in the United States,[29] and there has long been a need for more systematic research on the relationship of public health law infrastructure, agency effectiveness, and health outcomes.[30] COVID-19 produced considerable rapid research on specific health measures, but the empirical question of how various forms of authority affect outcomes is a matter of continuing importance in need of further, more rigorous study. Policy surveillance—the systematic, scientific tracking of laws of public health importance—provides data for evaluating changes in health authority.[31] Tracking changes and proposed changes in health law also enables stakeholders to recognize these changes and helps supporters of effective public health to weigh in. Finally, scientific legal mapping of proposed and enacted legislation can help distinguish political bluster and fringe legal proposals from those that actually become law.

Our research period ended before the conclusion of the legislative session or special sessions in the 2021–2022 legislative period. Bills that have been categorized as pending or vetoed in our study could still be enacted into law, as could new bills introduced after May 20, 2022.

Conclusions

COVID-19 posed a daunting challenge to health agencies everywhere. The transmissibility and adaptability of SARS-CoV-2 in a closely linked world explain much of the failure to prevent a global pandemic, but there were mistakes of both under- and overreaction. The ideal combination and timing of nonpharmaceutical interventions, and the best approaches to achieve high levels of vaccination, likely vary by setting and will be difficult to determine or sustain. Careful assessment of health agency performance and sensible revision of law are indicated.

Given the politicization of public health work during COVID-19 and the social shock of the pandemic, rapid and substantial changes to public health authority seem to reflect the frustration and irritation of a painful experience rather than a well-considered and evidence-informed analysis of the authority that health agencies need and what factors—leadership, funding, and other resources—drive strong health agency performance. Although restrictions specific to COVID-19 may not directly limit action in future emergencies, new legislation rarely seems to address the nuanced challenges of applying legal authority to stop pandemic disease. Rather, these laws appear to legislate a particular political position disdainful of public health and indifferent to the long-term dictates of effective public health practice.

Public Health Implications

The COVID-19 pandemic called for quick and decisive action to limit initial infections and subsequently a sustained effort to reduce transmission via nonpharmaceutical interventions and, when available, vaccines. When the next outbreak hits, new laws limiting health department discretion will make deploying these measures even more difficult. Now is the time for those concerned with effective public health action to focus on the basic law defining the scope, distribution, and nature of health authority. AJPH

ABOUT THE AUTHORS

All authors are with the Center for Public Health Law Research, Temple University Beasley School of Law, Philadelphia, PA.

CORRESPONDENCE

Correspondence should be sent to Katie Moran-McCabe, JD, 1719 N. Broad St, Room 509, Philadelphia, PA 19122 (e-mail: kathleen.mccabe@temple.edu). Reprints can be ordered at http://www.ajph.org by clicking the "Reprints" link.

PUBLICATION INFORMATION

Full Citation: Platt E, Moran-McCabe K, Cook A, Burris S. Trends in US state public health emergency laws, 2021–2022. *Am J Public Health*. 2023; 113(3):288–296.

Acceptance Date: December 18, 2022.

DOI: https://doi.org/10.2105/AJPH.2022.307214

CONTRIBUTORS

E. Platt led the project. E. Platt, K. Moran-McCabe, and S. Burris contributed substantially to the analysis and writing of the article. K. Moran-McCabe helped manage the project. A. Cook contributed substantially to the research.

ACKNOWLEDGMENTS

Support for this research was provided by the Robert Wood Johnson Foundation (awards 77249 and 79045).

Members of the following organizations provided assistance, guidance, or feedback in the research: ChangeLab Solutions, Network for Public Health Law, Public Health Law Center, Public Health Law Watch, the Association of State and Territorial Health Officials, and the Local Solutions Support Center. The authors thank Leslie Zellers for coordinating the collaborating teams. The authors thank Center for Public Health Law Research (CPHLR) staffers Adrienne Ghorashi and Lindsay Cloud, who provided guidance and assistance on this work, and Adam Herpolsheimer, Alexander Willhouse, Jonathan Larsen, Alexander Frazer, Caitlin Davie, DeAnna Baumle, Sterling Johnson, and Lindsey Gellar, who participated in building the data sets. The authors also thank Bethany Saxon and Hope Holroyd from CPHLR, who provided assistance with data visualization.

Note. The views expressed in this article do not necessarily reflect the views of the Robert Wood Johnson Foundation.

CONFLICTS OF INTEREST

The authors have no conflicts of interest to disclose.

HUMAN PARTICIPANT PROTECTION

No protocol approval was necessary because no human participants were involved in this study.

REFERENCES

1. Gostin LO, Burris S, Lazzarini Z. The law and the public's health: a study of infectious disease law in the United States. *Columbia Law Rev*. 1999; 99(1):59–128. https://doi.org/10.2307/1123597
2. Gostin LO, Wiley LF. *Public Health Law: Power, Duty, Restraint*. 3rd ed. Berkeley: University of California Press; 2016.
3. Burris S, de Guia S, Gable L, Levin D, Parmet WE, Terry NP. The legal response to COVID-19: legal pathways to a more effective and equitable response. *J Public Health Manag Pract*. 2021; 27(suppl 1):S72–S79. https://doi.org/10.1097/PHH.0000000000001277
4. Parmet WE, Khalik F. Judicial review of public health powers since the start of the COVID-19 pandemic: trends and implications. *Am J Public Health*. In press.
5. Anderson E, Tremper C, Thomas S, Wagenaar AC. Measuring statutory law and regulations for empirical research. In: Wagenaar A, Burris S, eds. *Public Health Law Research: Theory and Methods*. San Francisco: Wiley; 2013:237–260.
6. Gostin LO, Sapsin JW, Teret SP, et al. The Model State Emergency Health Powers Act: planning for and response to bioterrorism and naturally occurring infectious diseases. *JAMA*. 2002;288(5): 622–628. https://doi.org/10.1001/jama.288.5.622
7. Shaw FE, McKie KL, Liveoak CA, Goodman RA; State Public Health Counsel Review Team. Legal tools for preparedness and response: variation in quarantine powers among the 10 most populous US states in 2004. *Am J Public Health*. 2007; 97(suppl 1):S38–S43. https://doi.org/10.2105/AJPH.2005.083311
8. Guclu H, Ferrell Bjerke E, Galvan J, Sweeney P, Potter MA. State-level legal preparedness for nuclear and radiological emergencies in the US: a network analysis of state laws and regulations. *Public Health Rep*. 2014;129(suppl 4):154–165. https://doi.org/10.1177/00333549141296S420
9. Rothstein MA, Alcalde MG, Elster NR, et al. *Quarantine and Isolation: Lessons Learned From SARS: A Report to the Centers for Disease Control and Prevention*. Louisville, KY: Institute for Bioethics, Health Policy and Law; 2003.
10. Annas GJ. Bioterrorism, public health, and civil liberties. *N Engl J Med*. 2002;346(17):1337–1342. https://doi.org/10.1056/NEJM200204253461722
11. Richards EP, Rathbun KC. *Legislative Alternatives to the Model State Emergency Health Powers Act (MSEHPA)*. Baton Rouge, LA: LSU Program in Law, Science, and Public Health; 2003. White paper no. 2.
12. Network for Public Health Law. The Model State Emergency Health Powers Act: summary matrix. 2012. Available at: https://web.archive.org/web/20180722213558/https:/www.networkforphl.org/_asset/80p3y7/MSEHPA-States-Table-022812.pdf. Accessed August 8, 2022.
13. Erickson B. Limiting bill introductions. *LegisBriefs*. 2017;25(23). Available at: https://web.archive.org/web/20220929211235/https://www.ncsl.org/research/about-state-legislatures/limiting-bill-introductions.aspx. Accessed January 17, 2023.
14. LexisNexis. Why state legislative passage rates vary. 2020. Available at: https://www.lexisnexis.com/community/insights/legal/capitol-journal/b/state-net/posts/state-legislative-passage-rates. Accessed August 8, 2022.
15. Presley D, Burris S. *Comparing Federal Health Law Recommendations With State Health Legislation*. Philadelphia: Center for Public Health Law Research; 2014.
16. Goodman CB, Hatch ME, McDonald BD III. State preemption of local laws: origins and modern trends. *Perspect Public Manag Gov*. 2021;4(2): 146–158. https://doi.org/10.1093/ppmgov/gvaa018
17. Fowler L, Witt SL. State preemption of local authority: explaining patterns of state adoption of preemption measures. *Publius*. 2019;49(3):540–559.
18. Haddow K, Carr D, Winig BD, Adler S. Preemption, public health, and equity in the time of COVID-19. In: Burris S, de Guia S, Gable L, Levin DE, Parmet WE, Terry NP, eds. *COVID-19 Policy Playbook: Legal Recommendations for a Safer, More Equitable Future*. Boston: Public Health Law Watch; 2021:69–74.
19. Pomeranz JL, Silver D. State legislative strategies to pass, enhance, and obscure preemption of local public health policy-making. *Am J Prev Med*. 2020;59(3):333–342. https://doi.org/10.1016/j.amepre.2020.03.023
20. Carr D, Adler S, Winig BD, Montez JK. Equity first: conceptualizing a normative framework to assess the role of preemption in public health. *Milbank Q*. 2020;98(1):131–149. https://doi.org/10.1111/1468-0009.12444
21. Hodge JG Jr, Corbett A, Weidenaar K, Wetter SA. Public health "preemption plus." *J Law Med Ethics*. 2017;45(1):156–160. https://doi.org/10.1177/1073110517703110

22. Pomeranz JL, Pertschuk M. State preemption: a significant and quiet threat to public health in the United States. *Am J Public Health.* 2017;107(6):900–902. https://doi.org/10.2105/AJPH.2017.303756
23. Pertschuk M, Pomeranz JL, Aoki JR, Larkin MA, Paloma M. Assessing the impact of federal and state preemption in public health: a framework for decision makers. *J Public Health Manag Pract.* 2013;19(3):213–219. https://doi.org/10.1097/PHH.0b013e3182582a57
24. Wolf DA, Monnat SM, Montez JK. Effects of US state preemption laws on infant mortality. *Prev Med.* 2021;145:106417. https://doi.org/10.1016/j.ypmed.2021.106417
25. American Legislative Exchange Council. Emergency Power Limitation Act. 2021. Available at: https://alec.org/model-policy/emergency-power-limitation-act. Accessed November 18, 2022.
26. Montez JK, Beckfield J, Cooney JK, et al. US state policies, politics, and life expectancy. *Milbank Q.* 2020;98(3):668–699. https://doi.org/10.1111/1468-0009.12469
27. Gostin LO, Parmet WE, Rosenbaum S. The US Supreme Court's rulings on large business and health care worker vaccine mandates: ramifications for the COVID-19 response and the future of federal public health protection. *JAMA.* 2022;327(8):713–714. https://doi.org/10.1001/jama.2022.0852
28. Swindell D, Svara J, Stenberg C. Local government options in the era of state preemption. *LGR: Local Government Review.* July 2018. Available at: https://issuu.com/sdmunicipalleague/docs/9_sept_2018/s/14174881. Accessed January 7, 2023.
29. Anderson E, Burris S. Imagining a better public health (law) response to COVID-19. *Univ Richmond Law Rev.* 2022;56:955–1006.
30. Burris S, Mays GP, Douglas Scutchfield F, Ibrahim JK. Moving from intersection to integration: public health law research and public health systems and services research. *Milbank Q.* 2012;90(2):375–408. https://doi.org/10.1111/j.1468-0009.2012.00667.x
31. Burris S, Hitchcock L, Ibrahim JK, Penn M, Ramanathan T. Policy surveillance: a vital public health practice comes of age. *J Health Polit Policy Law.* 2016;41(6):1151–1167. https://doi.org/10.1215/03616878-3665931

Screening for and Experiences of Intimate Partner Violence in the United States Before, During, and After Pregnancy, 2016–2019

Katy B. Kozhimannil, PhD, MPA, Valerie A. Lewis, PhD, Julia D. Interrante, PhD, MPH, Phoebe L. Chastain, BA, and Lindsay Admon, MD, MSc

Objectives. To measure rates of intimate partner violence (IPV) screening during the perinatal period among people experiencing physical violence in the United States.

Methods. We used 2016–2019 Pregnancy Risk Assessment Monitoring System data (n = 158 338) to describe the incidence of physical IPV before or during pregnancy. We then assessed the prevalence of IPV screening before, during, or after pregnancy and predictors of receiving screening among those reporting violence.

Results. Among the 3.5% (n = 6259) of respondents experiencing violence, 58.7%, 26.9%, and 48.3% were not screened before, during, or after pregnancy, respectively. Those reporting Medicaid or no insurance at birth, American Indian/Alaska Native people, and Spanish-speaking Hispanic people faced increased risk of not having a health care visit during which screening might occur. Among those attending a health care visit, privately insured people, rural residents, and non-Hispanic White respondents faced increased risk of not being screened.

Conclusions. Among birthing people reporting physical IPV, nearly half were not screened for IPV before or after pregnancy. Public health efforts to improve maternal health must address both access to care and universal screening for IPV. (*Am J Public Health*. 2023;113(3):297–305. https://doi.org/10.2105/AJPH.2022.307195)

AJPH March 2023, Vol 113, No. 3

Maternal morbidity and mortality are increasing in the United States, with some individuals and communities experiencing disproportionate risk, including Black or American Indian/Alaska Native people, low-income individuals, and rural residents.[1–4] Many recent public health efforts addressing maternal mortality have focused on clinical risk factors and the quality of hospital-based care, but maternal safety outside the clinical setting, including in homes and communities, is equally important.[5,6]

Intimate partner violence (IPV) is a leading nonobstetric cause of maternal morbidity and mortality.[7–11] IPV includes physical, emotional, and sexual violence and comprises patterns of behavior to gain or maintain power and control.[12] Although physical violence is a commonly recognized form of IPV, emotional and sexual violence are also harmful and prevalent. Examples of emotional violence are verbal insults, humiliation, isolation from friends and family, threats of harm, controlling finances, and monitoring communication or location. Examples of sexual violence are forcing or attempting to force a partner to take part in a sex act, sexual touching, and nonphysical sexual events (e.g., sexting) when the partner does not or cannot consent.[13,14] Maternal experiences of IPV are associated with higher rates of preterm birth, lower birth weights, and lower rates of breastfeeding.[11,15] Risk of the most severe outcome, homicide perpetrated by an intimate partner, is heightened around the time of pregnancy and childbirth.[7,8,16–18] Approximately 60% of homicides that occur around the time of pregnancy are related to IPV.[7]

People who give birth frequently interact with clinicians before, during, and after pregnancy, making health care a crucial setting for IPV screening and intervention. Since 2012, the American College of Obstetricians and Gynecologists has recommended regular IPV screening during pregnancy and postpartum, and in 2018, the US Preventive Services Task Force upgraded their recommendation for IPV screening for reproductive-aged individuals from I (insufficient evidence) to B (recommended), supporting universal screening nationally.[19,20] Screening and referral to treatment may attenuate maternal and infant health inequities that are exacerbated by experiences of violence.[21] Still, IPV screening is not consistently provided for all reproductive age patients in either primary care or maternity services.[19,22,23]

Understanding the extent to which birthing people experience physical violence and whether they are screened for IPV before, during, and after pregnancy will provide critical insight for public health services and policy. We measured IPV screening during the perinatal period among those experiencing physical violence in a large representative sample of US residents who gave birth, and we discuss strategies to reduce the inequities identified.

METHODS

We used 2016–2019 data from 42 states and 2 jurisdictions (i.e., New York City and Washington, DC) from the Pregnancy Risk Assessment Monitoring System (PRAMS), conducted by the Centers for Disease Control and Prevention (CDC) in collaboration with state and city health departments.[24] We used PRAMS data from phase 8 surveys, which survey postpartum individuals between 2 and 6 months after childbirth. For each survey year, the CDC releases data that meet a minimum response rate threshold (55% in 2016–2017; 50% in 2018–2019).[24] Inclusion and exclusion criteria are described in Figure A (available as a supplement to the online version of this article at http://www.ajph.org).

Measures

Key outcome variables were (1) experiencing physical violence by a current or former intimate partner, and (2) screening for IPV at health care visits among those reporting physical violence.

The PRAMS survey asked whether a husband or partner or ex-husband or ex-partner pushed, hit, slapped, kicked, choked, or physically hurt the respondent in any other way. This outcome was coded as a dichotomous variable indicating whether the respondent reported experiencing physical violence, either before or during pregnancy.

Respondents were asked whether they had health care visits during the preconception period (12 months before pregnancy), prenatal care visits (during pregnancy), or any health care visits postpartum. If they reported a health care visit, they were asked whether a health care worker asked if someone was hurting them emotionally or physically. Although IPV comprises 3 types of violence (physical, emotional, and sexual), we described this as IPV screening, recognizing that respondents were asked about only 2 of the 3 potential aspects of IPV. Survey questions about screening were asked of individuals only about each respective period (preconception, pregnancy, postpartum) when they reported a health care visit, and we created a dichotomous indicator for screening for each of these periods among those reporting physical violence.

We selected the covariates included in our analyses a priori. Core sociodemographic variables were rural versus urban residency (based on National Center for Health Statistics Urban–Rural Classification Scheme for Counties),[25] race and ethnicity (non-Hispanic White, non-Hispanic Black, Hispanic [English-speaking and Spanish-speaking], American Indian/Alaska Native, Asian/Pacific Islander, and multiple/other), and health insurance status at childbirth (private insurance, Medicaid, and no insurance). Other sociodemographic variables were age (< 24, 25–34, and ≥ 35 years), education (< high school, high school, > high school), marital status (married and not married). We obtained the core and other sociodemographic variables from the linked birth certificate data. Clinical variables included parity, prepregnancy comorbidities (diabetes, high blood pressure/hypertension, depression, and smoking), and prepregnancy obesity, and we included them to account for the probability of greater health care interaction. We obtained parity from the birth certificate record, and all other clinical variables were reported in the PRAMS questionnaire.

Analysis

To describe characteristics of respondents who reported experiencing physical violence, we present survey-weighted proportions with 95% confidence intervals (CIs) using PRAMS weights, which account for the complex stratified survey design, and tested for distributional differences across characteristics by using the Rao–Scott χ^2 test.

Among respondents who reported physical violence, we used multivariate logistic regression to calculate adjusted predicted probabilities and percentage point risk differences (RDs). We calculated RDs using postestimation techniques available in Stata's margins command standardized to the distribution of covariates in the data. We calculated predicted probabilities and RDs of not attending a health care visit before, during, or after pregnancy—and thus not having an opportunity to be screened for IPV in the health care setting. Among those attending visits, we also calculated adjusted predicted probabilities and percentage point RDs for the lack of screening in each pregnancy period.

For each pregnancy period and each reason for not being screened, we calculated RDs across the core sociodemographic variables of rural versus urban residence, race and ethnicity, and health insurance status, comparing each to its reference category (i.e., urban, non-Hispanic White, and privately insured, respectively). We conducted several sensitivity analyses examining differences between respondents who did and those who did not report experiencing physical violence, predictors of not being screened among all birthing people, and predictors of not being screened prenatally across Kotelchuck Index levels of prenatal care adequacy to examine whether the number of prenatal visits could be associated with screening probability.[26]

We used Stata version 17.0 (StataCorp LLC, College Station, TX) and Stata's margins command in conducting analyses.

RESULTS

Physical violence before or during pregnancy was reported by 3.5% of this sample of US residents who gave birth between 2016 and 2019 (unweighted n = 6259/158 338; Table A, available as a supplement to the online version of this article at http://www.ajph.org). Compared with respondents who did not report physical violence, higher proportions of those who experienced physical violence were rural residents, identified as non-Hispanic Black or American Indian/Alaska Native, were younger, were less educated, were unmarried, were insured by Medicaid at childbirth, had a pregnancy that was unintended, and had higher proportions of clinical comorbidities ($P < .05$ for all comparisons described; Table A).

Table 1 shows the proportion of respondents with health care visits and IPV screening at visits for each pregnancy period among those who reported physical violence. During the 12 months before pregnancy, more than half of individuals who reported violence were not screened for IPV (58.7%; n = 3555/6259), either because they did not have a health care visit (32.9%; n = 2103/6259) or because they attended a visit but were not asked about abuse (38.4% of those experiencing physical violence who attended any visit; n = 1452/4156).

During pregnancy, almost all (98.2%; n = 6124) respondents who experienced physical violence reported having a prenatal care visit, so very few were not screened because of no prenatal care. However, 25.5% (n = 1326/6124) of those reporting prenatal care visits were not screened for IPV during any prenatal visit. As a result, 26.9% (n = 1461/6259) of those who experienced violence did not get screened at all during pregnancy.

Of respondents who experienced physical violence, 17% (n = 1196/6259) did not attend a postpartum health care visit. Of those who did, 62.4% (n = 3349/5063) were screened for IPV. As a result, 48.3% (n = 2910/6259) of postpartum people with a history of experiencing physical violence had no IPV screening after childbirth.

Among all birthing people, 65.7% were not screened for IPV before pregnancy, 29.7% were not screened during pregnancy, and 48.0% did not get screened during the postpartum period (Table B, available as a supplement to the online version of this article at http://www.ajph.org).

We examined associations between sociodemographic characteristics and IPV screening among respondents who reported physical violence, distinguishing between those who were not screened because they did not have a health care visit and those who were not screened at the visits they attended. Adjusted RDs for core characteristics (rural vs urban residency, race and ethnicity, and health insurance coverage at childbirth) are shown in Figures 1, 2, and 3, with specific percentage point differences reported in Table C (available as a supplement to the online version of this article at http://www.ajph.org). Table D (available as a supplement to the online version of this article at http://www.ajph.org) shows adjusted predicted probabilities of not receiving IPV screening by reason (i.e., no visit or not screened) overall and for each period (i.e., preconception, prenatal, and postpartum) among individuals who experienced physical violence with different sociodemographic characteristics.

Figure 1 shows adjusted differences in characteristics of those not screened for IPV in the preconception period by reason (i.e., no visit or not screened) among respondents who experienced physical violence. There were statistically significant differences by race and ethnicity, with a greater predicted proportion of Spanish-speaking Hispanic

TABLE 1— Health Care Visits and Intimate Partner Violence (IPV) Screening Among Patients Reporting Physical Violence: United States, Pregnancy Risk Assessment Monitoring System, 2016–2019

	Unweighted No. (Weighted %)	95% CI
Preconception		
Health care visit in the 12 mo before pregnancy		
No	2103 (32.9)	31.0, 34.9
Yes	4156 (67.1)	65.1, 69.1
If yes, received IPV screening		
No	1452 (38.4)	35.9, 41.0
Yes	2704 (61.6)	59.1, 64.1
Not screened (no visit or visit without screening)	3555 (58.7)	56.6, 60.7
Pregnancy		
Prenatal care visit		
No	135 (1.9)	1.4, 2.5
Yes	6124 (98.2)	97.5, 98.6
If yes, received IPV screening		
No	1326 (25.5)	23.6, 27.5
Yes	4798 (74.5)	72.5, 76.4
Not screened (no visit or visit without screening)	1461 (26.9)	25.0, 28.8
Postpartum		
Postpartum health care visit		
No	1196 (17.0)	15.6, 18.6
Yes	5063 (83.0)	81.4, 84.5
If yes, received IPV screening		
No	1714 (37.6)	35.4, 40.0
Yes	3349 (62.4)	60.0, 64.6
Not screened (no visit or visit without screening)	2910 (48.3)	46.2, 50.4

Note. CI = confidence interval. Sample size was n = 6259. Sample excludes 790 people who were younger than 18 years and not asked about violence/IPV and 3430 who had births in Vermont (which does not report race/ethnicity).

people who experienced physical violence (56.5%; Table D) not being screened because they lacked a health care visit in the 12 months before pregnancy compared with non-Hispanic White people (30.8%; Table D), with an adjusted difference of 25.7 percentage points (95% CI = 16.0, 35.3; Table C). By contrast, non-Hispanic White people reporting physical violence who were not screened at the preconception visits they attended (40.9%; Table D) constituted a higher predicted proportion compared with English-speaking Hispanic people (32.3%; an 8.5 percentage point difference; 95% CI = 0.8, 16.3; Tables C and D). People insured by Medicaid at childbirth and those without health insurance at childbirth, respectively, had a 9.6 (95% CI = 5.1, 14.2) and 22.6 (95% CI = 9.3, 35.9; Table C) percentage point higher probability of not having a health visit in the year before pregnancy compared with privately insured people (predicted proportions = 34.7%, 47.7%, and 25.1%, respectively; Table D). However, people with private insurance at childbirth had a 6.9 percentage point (95% CI = 0.7, 13.1; Table C) higher probability of not being screened for IPV at the visits they attended compared with those with Medicaid coverage (43.0% and 36.1%, respectively; Table D).

Figure 2 focuses on pregnancy and shows adjusted differences in characteristics of those who experienced physical violence and did not receive IPV screening, either because they did not have a prenatal care visit or because they were not screened at the visits they attended. More than 90% of respondents reporting physical violence attended at least 1 prenatal visit, so differences were concentrated among those who attended a visit but were not screened for abuse.

Groups at increased risk for not being screened included rural residents and privately insured people, with adjusted differences of 7.2 percentage points (rural vs urban; 95% CI = 2.1, 12.4) and 7.8 percentage points (private insurance vs Medicaid; 95% CI = 3.1, 12.6; Table C). Additionally, adjusted RDs for screening among non-Hispanic Black and American Indian/Alaska Native survivors were 6.1 percentage points (95% CI = 1.0, 11.3) and 10.0 percentage points (95% CI = 2.0, 18.0) higher, respectively, than rates for non-Hispanic White people who experienced physical violence (Table C). Among people experiencing physical violence who were rural residents, non-Hispanic White, or privately insured, the predicted proportions not screened during prenatal care were 31.0%, 27.4%, and 31.0%, respectively (Table D). Differences in screening by the adequacy of prenatal care were inconsistent across sociodemographic characteristics examined, as shown in Table E (available as a supplement to the online version of this article at http://www.ajph.org).

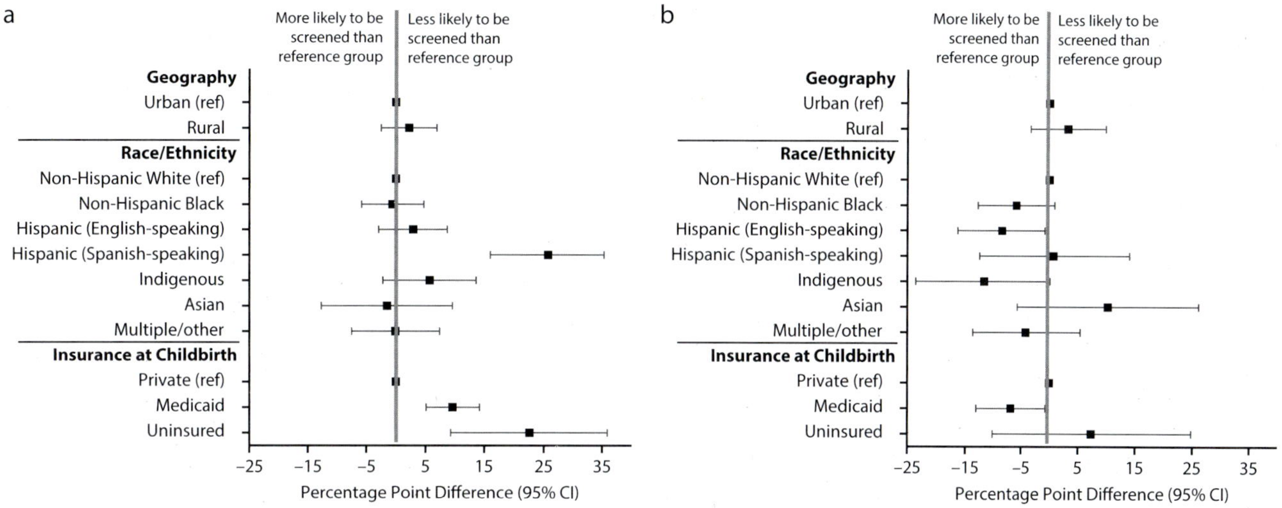

FIGURE 1— Adjusted Differences in Characteristics of Patients Not Receiving Intimate Partner Violence Screening in the Preconception Period Among Patients Reporting Physical Violence Who (a) Were Not Screened Because of No Visit, and (b) Visited but Were Not Screened: United States, Pregnancy Risk Assessment Monitoring System, 2016–2019

Note. CI = confidence interval. The sample size was n = 6259. Model also adjusted for maternal age, education, marital status, parity, and prepregnancy conditions (obesity, diabetes, high blood pressure/hypertension, smoking, or depression). Percentage point difference estimates were based on multivariable logistic regression results. Values for percentage point differences are provided in Table C (available as a supplement to the online version of this article at http://www.ajph.org). Adjusted predicted probability values from which differences were calculated are provided in Table D (available as a supplement to the online version of this article at http://www.ajph.org).

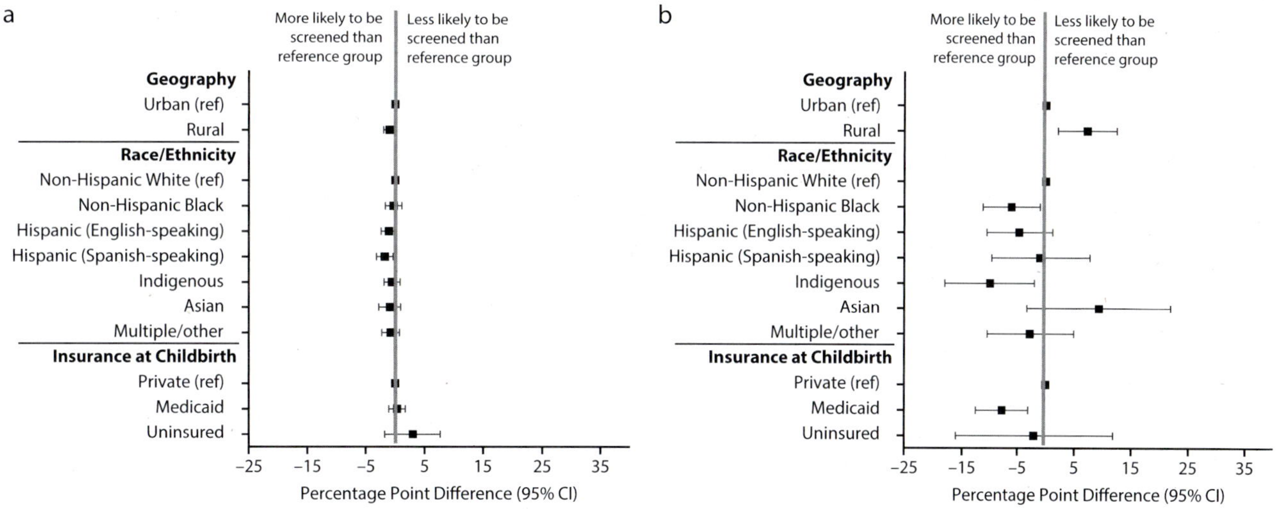

FIGURE 2— Adjusted Differences in Characteristics of Patients Not Receiving Intimate Partner Violence Screening During Pregnancy Among Patients Reporting Physical Violence Who (a) Were Not Screened Because of No Visit, and (b) Visited but Were Not Screened: United States, Pregnancy Risk Assessment Monitoring System, 2016–2019

Note. CI = confidence interval. The sample size was n = 6259. The model also adjusted for maternal age, education, marital status, parity, and prepregnancy conditions (obesity, diabetes, high blood pressure/hypertension, smoking, or depression). Percentage point difference estimates were based on multivariable logistic regression results. Values for percentage point differences are provided in Table C (available as a supplement to the online version of this article at http://www.ajph.org). Adjusted predicted probability values from which differences were calculated are provided in Table D (available as a supplement to the online version of this article at http://www.ajph.org).

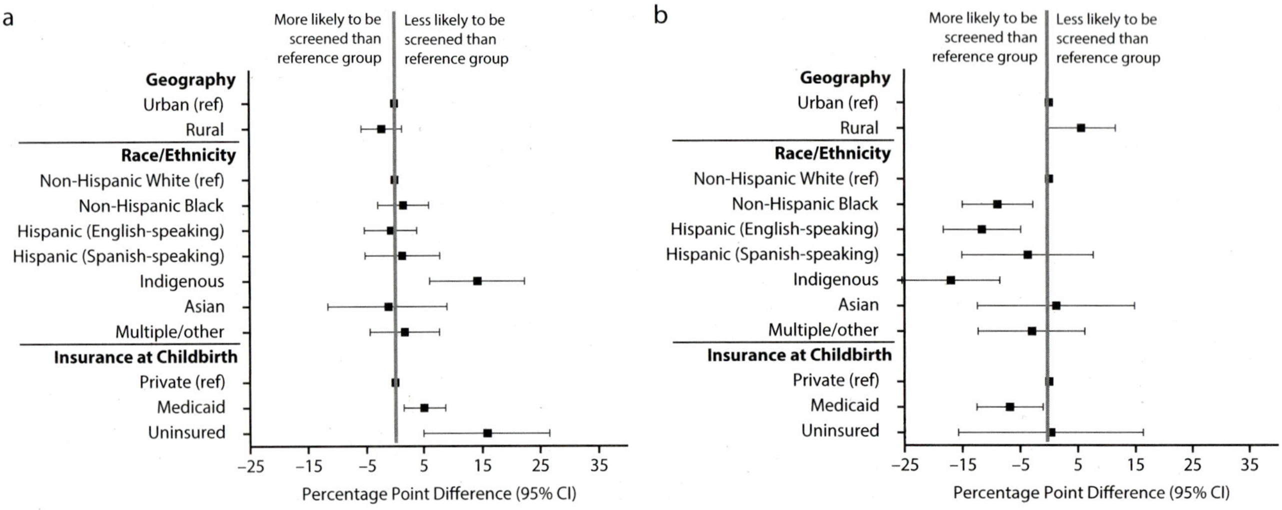

FIGURE 3— Adjusted Differences in Characteristics of Patients Not Receiving Intimate Partner Violence Screening in the Postpartum Period Among Patients Reporting Physical Violence Who (a) Were Not Screened Because of No Visit, and (b) Visited but Were Not Screened: United States, Pregnancy Risk Assessment Monitoring System, 2016–2019

Note. CI = confidence interval. The sample size was n = 6259. The model also adjusted for maternal age, education, marital status, parity, and prepregnancy conditions (obesity, diabetes, high blood pressure/hypertension, smoking, or depression). Percentage point difference estimates were based on multivariable logistic regression results. Values for percentage point differences are provided in Table C (available as a supplement to the online version of this article at http://www.ajph.org). Adjusted predicted probability values from which differences were calculated are provided in Table D (available as a supplement to the online version of this article at http://www.ajph.org).

IPV screening in the postpartum period is the focus in Figure 3. Among those who experienced physical violence, there were large differences by race and ethnicity and by insurance status in lacking postpartum visits, with American Indian/Alaska Native people 14.2 percentage points (95% CI = 6.1, 22.3; Table C) more likely than non-Hispanic White people to not have a postpartum visit where screening could occur (30.1% and 15.9%, respectively; Table D). Additionally, people with Medicaid coverage at childbirth (17.5%) and those without insurance at childbirth (28.1%) experiencing physical violence were at elevated risk for not having postpartum care compared with those with private insurance (12.3%; percentage point differences = 5.1; 95% CI = 1.5, 8.8 and 15.8; 95% CI = 5.0, 26.6; Table C).

Among those reporting physical violence who did have a visit postpartum, non-Hispanic White people and privately insured people had elevated predicted proportions not screened for IPV at postpartum visits (41.5% and 42.4%, respectively; Table D). Although a higher proportion of American Indian/Alaska Native (vs non-Hispanic White) people did not have a postpartum visit, those that did receive care after childbirth had a 17.0 percentage point (95% CI = 25.4, 8.5; Table C) higher probability than did non-Hispanic White people of being screened for abuse at the visit they attended.

DISCUSSION

IPV is a risk factor for maternal morbidity and mortality, and homicide is a leading cause of death during pregnancy and postpartum.[10] Our analysis indicated that 3.5% of birthing people in this study reported physical violence in the context of IPV. This equates to approximately 280 000 people who gave birth between 2016 and 2019 in 42 states and 2 US jurisdictions who reported being pushed, hit, slapped, kicked, choked, or otherwise physically hurt by current or former intimate partners. Of these, we found that more than half (58.7%) were not screened for IPV before pregnancy, more than a quarter (26.9%) lacked screening during pregnancy, and nearly half (48.3%) were not screened postpartum, either because they did not have a health care visit during these periods or because they attended a visit but were not asked whether someone had hurt them physically or emotionally. These individuals are a critically at-risk population for whom targeted clinical and policy interventions may be important and impactful.

Our analysis revealed 2 distinct reasons that people experiencing IPV around the time of pregnancy were not screened. The first reason is lack of perinatal health care visits. Spanish-speaking Hispanic people, American

Indian/Alaska Native people, those with Medicaid at childbirth, and people without insurance at childbirth were less likely than were non-Hispanic White and privately insured people to attend preconception and postpartum visits at which IPV screening could occur. Focusing on access to care in these populations may increase opportunities for IPV screening.

The second reason is lack of screening at health care visits attended by respondents. Among those experiencing physical violence and attending health care visits, rural (vs urban) residents, non-Hispanic White (vs racialized) people, and those with private insurance (vs Medicaid or no insurance) were less likely to be screened during their encounters with the health care system. Those overlooked for screening may reflect clinicians' perceptions about who is at risk for physical, emotional, or sexual violence. Additionally, health care systems and practices caring for more advantaged individuals (e.g., non-Hispanic White, privately insured) are less likely to include IPV screening in routinized care.[27]

Non-Hispanic Black and American Indian/Alaska Native individuals experience the highest rates of IPV-associated homicide compared with other racial groups,[4] and pregnancy exacerbates this racialized pattern of harm.[28] Our analysis indicated risks of potential underdetection among Spanish-speaking Hispanic people (before pregnancy) and American Indian/Alaska Native people (during the postpartum period) who reported physical violence by a current or former intimate partner.

Clinical and Policy Implications

Clinical and policy organizations recommend universal IPV screening and referral to support services to increase the safety of survivors and their families and to address health risks.[29] These findings indicate that the US health care system falls short on universal IPV screening during a critical period in the life course. Efforts to improve screening rates could include changes to reimbursement or financing for IPV screening, such as requiring managed care organizations or hospitals that contract with state Medicaid programs or that receive matching federal funds to implement routine screening as a condition of payment. Similar financial policy interventions have been successful in reducing rates of early elective delivery at the time of childbirth and improving maternity care quality generally.[30,31]

Improving access to perinatal health care visits, including assessing how visit attendance may be affected by IPV, is an important area for research and policy intervention. We found that people experiencing physical abuse who had Medicaid coverage at childbirth as well as those who were uninsured when they gave birth had higher risks than did privately insured people of not receiving a health care visit in the year before pregnancy or having a postpartum follow-up visit. Access to care influences service use and screening in the perinatal period, and efforts to improve access to care through Medicaid expansion and postpartum insurance eligibility extensions could improve IPV screening in the perinatal period.[32,33]

Improving the frequency and efficacy of screening may require investment in trauma-informed, evidence-based training for clinicians who interact with patients around the time of pregnancy. These include a variety of health professions—obstetricians, family physicians, midwives, psychologists, psychiatrists, licensed family and marriage therapists, social workers, substance abuse and addiction specialists, nurses, nurse practitioners, physician assistants, pediatricians, maternal–fetal medicine specialists, neonatologists, and emergency physicians—as well as nonclinical staff. IPV takes many forms and is not limited to physical violence, yet clinician training and understanding of the multiple complex facets of IPV are often limited.[34] Our findings highlight the importance of ensuring universal screening among those attending health care visits and addressing potential clinician bias about who is at risk for experiencing IPV.

Additionally, efforts to ensure the availability of referral and treatment of patients who screen positive for IPV, as well as providing support to both clinicians and patients who interact with systems outside health care in the context of IPV, are essential to promote patient safety and well-being.

Limitations

This study has several important limitations. Respondents were not asked about experiences of emotional or sexual violence, likely resulting in an underestimate of the true prevalence of IPV, as study respondents were asked only about experiences of physical violence. Similarly, the question about screening for IPV did not encompass sexual violence. Survey questions in the PRAMS data and other surveillance efforts could be improved to better measure IPV. Self-reported physical violence and IPV screening are both subject to potential biases. Physical violence is underdetected and underreported, generally because of social desirability bias, and may be differentially underreported by characteristics of interest, including race and ethnicity, rural versus urban residency, and health insurance status.[21] Additionally, in the PRAMS data, experiences of violence are not asked about during the postpartum period. Self-reports of screening may be affected by recall bias (i.e., whether a respondent remembers being screened), which could be related to the results of the screening.[15]

The generalizability of this study is limited, as results do not represent the experiences of people who gave birth in 7 US states (i.e., Arizona, California, Idaho, Nevada, Ohio, South Carolina, and Texas). The postpartum visit rate of PRAMS respondents is higher than the national average, and response rates are higher among non-Hispanic White and socioeconomically advantaged groups, so estimates of physical violence and IPV screening may be differentially conservative based on patient characteristics.[24,35]

Conclusions

As rates of US maternal morbidity and mortality increase, the role of IPV has become increasingly clear. Approximately half of birthing people who reported physical violence before or during pregnancy were not screened because they did not have a health care visit in the year before pregnancy or postpartum or because they were not screened for IPV at the visits they attended. Among those who experienced IPV, we found that Spanish-speaking Hispanic and American Indian/Alaska Native people and those with Medicaid coverage or no health insurance at childbirth were at greater risk for being unscreened than were non-Hispanic White and privately insured people because of lack of visits.

Additionally, some birthing people experiencing physical violence—including those who were non-Hispanic White rural residents and those who were privately insured at childbirth—were at higher risk for not being screened at the visits they attended than were racialized, urban, or uninsured people or those with Medicaid who experienced violence and attended visits. These findings imply a critical need for increased health care access and better screening to identify and support people experiencing violence by an intimate partner. More broadly, clinical and policy efforts to improve maternal health in the United States should address IPV as a public health policy issue. AJPH

ABOUT THE AUTHORS

Katy B. Kozhimannil, Julia D. Interrante, and Phoebe L. Chastain are with the University of Minnesota School of Public Health, Minneapolis. Valerie A. Lewis is with the University of North Carolina at Chapel Hill. Lindsay Admon is with the University of Michigan Institute for Healthcare Policy and Innovation, Ann Arbor.

CORRESPONDENCE

Correspondence should be sent to Katy Backes Kozhimannil, PhD, MPA, University of Minnesota School of Public Health, Division of Health Policy and Management, 420 Delaware St SE, MMC 729, Minneapolis, MN 55455 (e-mail: kbk@umn.edu). Reprints can be ordered at http://www.ajph.org by clicking the "Reprints" link.

PUBLICATION INFORMATION

Full Citation: Kozhimannil KB, Lewis VA, Interrante JD, Chastain PL, Admon L. Screening for and experiences of intimate partner violence in the United States before, during, and after pregnancy, 2016–2019. *Am J Public Health*. 2023;113(3):297–305.

Acceptance Date: December 5, 2022.

DOI: https://doi.org/10.2105/AJPH.2022.307195

CONTRIBUTORS

K. B. Kozhimannil led data interpretation and oversaw the study. K. B. Kozhimannil and V. A. Lewis conceptualized and designed the study. K. B. Kozhimannil, V. A. Lewis, and J. D. Interrante drafted portions of the article. J. D. Interrante led the statistical analysis. V. A. Lewis, J. D. Interrante, P. L. Chastain, and L. Admon contributed to study design and data interpretation and revised the article. L. Admon acquired the study data.

ACKNOWLEDGMENTS

This research was supported in part by the National Institutes of Health (NIH), National Center for Advancing Translational Sciences (grant UL1TR002494). L. Admon is supported by the Agency for Healthcare Research and Quality (grant K08HS027640) and the NIH (grants R01MH120124 and R01MD014958).

The authors gratefully acknowledge all Pregnancy Risk Surveillance and Monitoring System (PRAMS) study participants and members of the PRAMS Working Group at the Centers for Disease Control and Prevention. The authors also thank Alyssa H. Fritz, MPH, RD, for helpful input on the article.

Note. The content is solely the responsibility of the authors and does not necessarily represent the official views of the Agency for Healthcare Research and Quality or the NIH.

CONFLICTS OF INTEREST

The authors have no conflicts of interest to disclose.

HUMAN PARTICIPANT PROTECTION

Data were de-identified, and this study was designated exempt from review by the University of Michigan's and the University of Minnesota's institutional review boards.

REFERENCES

1. Joseph KS, Boutin A, Lisonkova S, et al. Maternal mortality in the United States: recent trends, current status, and future considerations. *Obstet Gynecol.* 2021;137(5):763–771. https://doi.org/10.1097/AOG.0000000000004361
2. Hoyert DL. Maternal mortality rates in the United States, 2020. February 2022. Available at: https://www.cdc.gov/nchs/data/hestat/maternal-mortality/2020/E-stat-Maternal-Mortality-Rates-2022.pdf. Accessed October 7, 2022.
3. Taylor J, Novoa C, Hamm K, Phadke S. Eliminating racial disparities in maternal and infant mortality. May 2, 2019. Available at: https://www.americanprogress.org/article/eliminating-racial-disparities-maternal-infant-mortality. Accessed October 7, 2022.
4. Centers for Disease Control and Prevention. Racial and ethnic differences in homicides of adult women and the role of intimate partner violence—United States, 2003–2014. *MMWR Morb Mortal Wkly Rep.* 2017;66(28):741–746. https://doi.org/10.15585/mmwr.mm6628a1
5. Wang E, Glazer KB, Howell EA, Janevic TM. Social determinants of pregnancy-related mortality and morbidity in the United States: a systematic review. *Obstet Gynecol.* 2020;135(4):896–915. https://doi.org/10.1097/AOG.0000000000003762
6. Crear-Perry J, Correa-de-Araujo R, Lewis Johnson T, McLemore MR, Neilson E, Wallace M. Social and structural determinants of health inequities in maternal health. *J Womens Health (Larchmt).* 2021;30(2):230–235. https://doi.org/10.1089/jwh.2020.8882
7. Wallace ME, Friar N, Herwehe J, Theall KP. Violence as a direct cause of and indirect contributor to maternal death. *J Womens Health (Larchmt).*

2020;29(8):1032–1038. https://doi.org/10.1089/jwh.2019.8072

8. Campbell J, Matoff-Stepp S, Velez ML, Cox HH, Laughon K. Pregnancy-associated deaths from homicide, suicide, and drug overdose: review of research and the intersection with intimate partner violence. *J Womens Health (Larchmt)*. 2021;30(2):236–244. https://doi.org/10.1089/jwh.2020.8875
9. Alhusen JL, Ray E, Sharps P, Bullock L. Intimate partner violence during pregnancy: maternal and neonatal outcomes. *J Womens Health (Larchmt)*. 2015;24(1):100–106. https://doi.org/10.1089/jwh.2014.4872
10. Wallace M, Gillispie-Bell V, Cruz K, Davis K, Vilda D. Homicide during pregnancy and the postpartum period in the United States, 2018–2019. *Obstet Gynecol*. 2021;138(5):762–769. [Erratum in: *Obstet Gynecol*. 2022;139(2):347]. https://doi.org/10.1097/AOG.0000000000004567
11. Gartland D, Hemphill SA, Hegarty K, Brown SJ. Intimate partner violence during pregnancy and the first year postpartum in an Australian pregnancy cohort study. *Matern Child Health J*. 2011;15(5):570–578. https://doi.org/10.1007/s10995-010-0638-z
12. United Nations. Domestic abuse: how to respond? Available at: https://www.un.org/en/coronavirus/domestic-abuse. Accessed October 7, 2022.
13. Pence E, Paymar M. *Education Groups for Men Who Batter: The Duluth Model*. New York, NY: Springer; 1993.
14. Havard TE, Lefevre M. Beyond the power and control wheel: how abusive men manipulate mobile phone technologies to facilitate coercive control. *J Gend Based Violence*. 2020;4(2):223–239. https://doi.org/10.1332/239868020X15850131608789
15. Chaves K, Eastwood J, Ogbo FA, et al. Intimate partner violence identified through routine antenatal screening and maternal and perinatal health outcomes. *BMC Pregnancy Childbirth*. 2019;19(1):357. https://doi.org/10.1186/s12884-019-2527-9
16. Wallace ME, Crear-Perry J, Mehta PK, Theall KP. Homicide during pregnancy and the postpartum period in Louisiana, 2016–2017. *JAMA Pediatr*. 2020;174(4):387–388. [Erratum in: *JAMA Pediatr*. 2020;174(4):393]. https://doi.org/10.1001/jamapediatrics.2019.5853.
17. Miller JM, Rensing S. Integrating national violent death reporting system data into maternal mortality review committees. *J Womens Health (Larchmt)*. 2021;30(11):1573–1579. https://doi.org/10.1089/jwh.2021.0058
18. Strand SJM, Storey JE. Intimate partner violence in urban, rural, and remote areas: an investigation of offense severity and risk factors. *Violence Against Women*. 2019;25(2):188–207. https://doi.org/10.1177/1077801218766611
19. ACOG Committee opinion no. 518: intimate partner violence. *Obstet Gynecol*. 2012;119(2, pt 1):412–417. https://doi.org/10.1097/AOG.0b013e318249ff74
20. US Preventive Services Task Force. Screening for intimate partner violence, elder abuse, and abuse of vulnerable adults: US Preventive Services Task Force final recommendation statement. *JAMA*. 2018;320(16):1678–1687. https://doi.org/10.1001/jama.2018.14741
21. O'Doherty L, Hegarty K, Ramsay J, Davidson LL, Feder G, Taft A. Screening women for intimate partner violence in healthcare settings. *Cochrane Database Syst Rev*. 2015;2015(7):CD007007. https://doi.org/10.1002/14651858.CD007007.pub3
22. Kapaya M, Boulet SL, Warner L, Harrison L, Fowler D. Intimate partner violence before and during pregnancy, and prenatal counseling among women with a recent live birth, United States, 2009–2015. *J Womens Health (Larchmt)*. 2019;28(11):1476–1486. https://doi.org/10.1089/jwh.2018.7545
23. Kalra N, Hooker L, Reisenhofer S, Di Tanna GL, García-Moreno C. Training healthcare providers to respond to intimate partner violence against women. *Cochrane Database Syst Rev*. 2021;5(5):CD012423. https://doi.org/10.1002/14651858.CD012423.pub2
24. Shulman HB, D'Angelo DV, Harrison L, Smith RA, Warner L. The Pregnancy Risk Assessment Monitoring System (PRAMS): overview of design and methodology. *Am J Public Health*. 2018;108(10):1305–1313. https://doi.org/10.2105/AJPH.2018.304563
25. Centers for Disease Control and Prevention. NCHS urban–rural classification scheme for counties. December 2, 2019. Available at: https://www.cdc.gov/nchs/data_access/urban_rural.htm. Accessed October 7, 2022.
26. Kotelchuck M. The adequacy of prenatal care utilization index: its US distribution and association with low birthweight. *Am J Public Health*. 1994;84(9):1486–1489. https://doi.org/10.2105/ajph.84.9.1486
27. Fraze TK, Brewster AL, Lewis VA, Beidler LB, Murray GF, Colla CH. Prevalence of screening for food insecurity, housing instability, utility needs, transportation needs, and interpersonal violence by US physician practices and hospitals. *JAMA Netw Open*. 2019;2(9):e1911514. https://doi.org/10.1001/jamanetworkopen.2019.11514
28. Kivisto AJ, Mills S, Elwood LS. Racial disparities in pregnancy-associated intimate partner homicide. *J Interpers Violence*. 2022;37(13–14):NP10938–NP10961. https://doi.org/10.1177/0886260521990831
29. Koch AR, Geller SE. Addressing maternal deaths due to violence: the Illinois experience. *Am J Obstet Gynecol*. 2017;217(5):556.e1–556.e6. https://doi.org/10.1016/j.ajog.2017.08.005
30. Washio Y, Atreyapurapu S, Hayashi Y, et al. Systematic review on use of health incentives in U.S. to change maternal health behavior. *Prev Med*. 2021;145:106442. https://doi.org/10.1016/j.ypmed.2021.106442
31. Fowler TT, Schiff J, Applegate MS, Griffith K, Fairbrother GL. Early elective deliveries accounted for nearly 9 percent of births paid for by Medicaid. *Health Aff (Millwood)*. 2014;33(12):2170–2178. https://doi.org/10.1377/hlthaff.2014.0534
32. Bellerose M, Collin L, Daw JR. The ACA Medicaid expansion and perinatal insurance, health care use, and health outcomes: a systematic review. *Health Aff (Millwood)*. 2022;41(1):60–68. https://doi.org/10.1377/hlthaff.2021.01150
33. Admon LK, Daw JR, Winkelman TNA, et al. Insurance coverage and perinatal health care use among low-income women in the US, 2015–2017. *JAMA Netw Open*. 2021;4(1):e2034549. https://doi.org/10.1001/jamanetworkopen.2020.34549
34. Bonomi AE. Preventing violence-related maternal death: a call to action. *J Womens Health (Larchmt)*. 2020;29(8):1021–1022. https://doi.org/10.1089/jwh.2020.8415
35. Hebert LE, Sarche MC. Pre-pregnancy and prenatal alcohol use among American Indian and Alaska Native and Non-Hispanic White women: findings from PRAMS in five states. *Matern Child Health J*. 2021;25(9):1392–1401. https://doi.org/10.1007/s10995-021-03159-7

Economic Empowerment, HIV Risk Behavior, and Mental Health Among School-Going Adolescent Girls in Uganda: Longitudinal Cluster-Randomized Controlled Trial, 2017–2022

Fred M. Ssewamala, PhD, Rachel Brathwaite, PhD, and Torsten B. Neilands, PhD

See also Baumann and Devkota, p. 246.

AJPH March 2023, Vol 113, No. 3

Objectives. To investigate the long-term (12- and 24-month) impact of an economic empowerment intervention on HIV risk behaviors and mental health among school-going adolescent girls in Uganda.

Methods. A total of 1260 girls aged 14 to 17 years were randomized at the school level to (1) standard health and sex education (controls; n = 408 students; n = 16 schools), (2) 1-to-1 matched savings youth development account (YDA; n = 471 students; n = 16 schools), or (3) combination intervention (YDA and multiple family group [YDA+MFG]; n = 15 schools; n = 381 students). Mixed-effects models were fitted.

Results. YDA and YDA+MFG girls had significantly lower depressive symptoms and better self-concept than controls at 24 months. Only YDA+MFG girls had significantly lower hopelessness levels than controls. There were no significant study group differences at 12 and 24 months for sexual risk-taking behavior and attitudes. There was no significant difference between YDA and YDA+MFG groups for all outcomes.

Conclusions. Providing YDA and MFG can positively improve adolescent girls' mental health, but our analyses showed no significant differences across groups on sexual risk-taking behaviors. Future studies may consider replicating these interventions and analyses in older populations, including those transitioning into young adults.

Trial Registration. ClinicalTrials.gov Identifier: NCT03307226. (*Am J Public Health*. 2023;113(3):306–315. https://doi.org/10.2105/AJPH.2022.307169)

Approximately 90% of all adolescents living with HIV worldwide reside in the resource-limited region of sub-Saharan Africa (SSA).[1] However, the majority (70%) of new HIV infections among youths aged 15 to 19 years occur among adolescent girls.[2] The SSA region also has a substantial burden of mental health problems among adolescents,[3] and research shows that girls have a disproportionately higher burden of mental health problems than boys.[4,5] Girls often report significantly worse internalizing disorders (reflective of the child's psychological and emotional state) than boys, and this gender gap increases with age.[6] As a consequence, adolescent girls represent an important vulnerable population at increased risk of HIV infection[7] and poor mental health in SSA. Therefore, interventions designed for adolescent girls in SSA should innovatively address both HIV risk reduction and adolescent mental health because they can contribute to curbing the spread of the HIV epidemic[8] and preventing progression of poor health and social problems in adulthood.

In Uganda, a resource-limited SSA country extensively affected by the HIV epidemic, approximately 800 000 girls and women are living with HIV.[9] Poverty is a major factor that increases adolescent girls' risk for HIV infection and transmission. More than half (56%) of adolescents in Uganda are exposed to multidimensional poverty and low living standards.[10]

Sociocultural norms and beliefs present in Ugandan communities often influence decision-making, and in scenarios where there are limited financial resources, female children are often excluded from educational opportunities, favoring male children instead.[11] Financial insecurity drastically reduces families' ability to send girls to school where vital education on HIV/AIDS prevention and access to psychosocial support and health and medical services is received.[12]

Indeed, out-of-school girls have increased vulnerability to HIV infection[13] as they are forced to engage in risk-taking activities to improve their financial security. In Uganda, out-of-school girls are particularly vulnerable to transactional sex with older men, unprotected sex, early sexual initiation, early marriage, and adolescent pregnancy, which all heighten their risk of infection with HIV and other sexually transmitted infections (STIs).[14,15] For those reasons, it is important to intervene with adolescent girls while they are still in school, to keep them in school.

Poverty is also a significant risk factor for the development and persistence of poor mental health. In the resource-limited region of SSA, there are inadequate numbers of qualified mental health professionals to diagnose and treat mental health conditions and disproportionate distribution of human resources between urban and rural areas. For example, for every 100 000 people that may need a mental health professional, there are 0.08 qualified psychiatrists.[16] Moreover, only 1% of Uganda's gross domestic product is allocated to mental health care, which is inclusive of services for children, adolescents, and adults.[16] Poverty-impacted communities significantly perpetuate poor mental health because there are often high levels of environmental stressors, lack of social support, violence against children, high unemployment, food insecurity, and other social and health problems that are all risk factors for children's and adolescents' poor mental health.[17,18]

Adolescence is a period marked by increased vulnerability to mental and substance-use disorders,[19] and there are concerns that early sexual debut often results in sexual risk-taking (i.e. inconsistent condom use, unsafe sex, multiple sexual partners), making one vulnerable to acquiring HIV.[20–22] Furthermore, living with HIV as a chronic, highly stigmatized, and transmittable illness can increase one's risk of poor mental health.[23] Hence, extra attention should be placed on adolescent girls in low-resource SSA communities who are already vulnerable given their economic disadvantage.

Research on effective evidence-based interventions to prevent poor mental health and reduce HIV risk among adolescent girls residing in Uganda and other resource-limited SSA countries are lacking.[24] The Suubi4Her study was designed to help fill this gap while simultaneously addressing the main underlying risk factors for HIV risk and poor mental health among adolescent girls in Uganda.[25] Suubi4Her is a 3-arm cluster-randomized controlled trial designed to reduce HIV risk behaviors and improve mental health among adolescent girls across 47 public secondary schools in Uganda.

Given the economic factors driving HIV risk and poor mental health among adolescents in low-resource communities, the interventions implemented in the Suubi4Her study are guided by asset theory.[26,27] Asset theory posits that individuals with financial assets have improved economic security and report psychological benefits such as future-oriented thinking, feelings of self-efficacy, and security. Thus, girls in the intervention arms of the Suubi4Her study received youth development accounts (YDAs), 1-to-1 matched savings accounts. The matched funds can be used to pay for girls' education and skills training fees (up to 70%) or family-based income-generating activities (up to 30% of matched savings). All participants received training on principles of financial management, which covered saving, asset-building, using financial institutions, and income generation.

Furthermore, because families residing in deprived communities are likely to experience high stress, lack of social support, and social isolation, which all negatively influence parenting and family relationships,[28] the Suubi4Her study also incorporated multiple family groups (MFGs) as an intervention. MFGs aim to strengthen family communication and reduce stigma by providing a safe space for parents and children to communicate with themselves and other families.[29] Research showed that good parent–child relationships and frequent and open communication (including about sex) between children and their caregivers (especially mothers) is associated with later sexual debut and less engagement in risk behaviors.[30–32] As such, adolescent girls in the second intervention arm received a combination intervention comprising YDAs plus MFGs (YDA+MFG).

In this study, we investigated the long-term impact of the Suubi4Her intervention on HIV risk behaviors (i.e., sexual risk-taking) and mental health (depressive symptoms, hopelessness, self-esteem, and self-concept) among school-going adolescent girls. We hypothesized that (1) girls in the YDA group would have better mental health outcomes and less sexual risk-taking behaviors than those in the control condition, (2) girls in the YDA+MFG group will show better mental health and less sexual risk-taking behaviors than counterparts in the control condition, and (3) girls in the YDA+MFG group would have better outcomes than their counterparts in the YDA group alone.

METHODS

The Suubi4her study is a longitudinal 3-arm cluster-randomized controlled trial conducted in 47 public secondary schools in the central region of Uganda (Rakai, Kyotera, Masaka, Lwengo, and Kalungu districts; 2017–2022).[25] This region has a heavy burden of HIV (prevalence of 10.6% vs 7.4% in Uganda).[33] This is also a geographically stable region with infrequent migration, enabling easy tracking of participants over the study period.

A total of 1260 adolescent girls aged 14 to 17 years were enrolled and followed up at 12 and 24 months (Appendix, Figure A, available as a supplement to the online version of this article at https://ajph.org). To reduce contamination, randomization was done at the school level to 1 of 3 study conditions. The first condition was a usual care or control arm that received standard health and sex education (n = 16 schools; n = 408 students). All girls in each study group received this standard health and sex education component. In Uganda, this is a mandatory curriculum authorized by the Ministry of Education, which covers adolescent sexual and reproductive health. Topics included delaying sex, using condoms and contraception, preventing forced sex, preventing substance use, gender equality, and importance of delaying marriage.

The second condition was treatment arm 1: YDA. Each participant was enrolled in a 1-to-1 match rate savings program (n = 16 schools; n = 471 students). The third condition was treatment arm 2: participants received a combination intervention composed of YDA and an evidence-based family strengthening intervention designed to enhance youth behavioral health delivered using an MFG format (YDA+MFG; n = 15 schools; n = 381 students; Appendix, pages 1–3 and Table A).

Within each school, adolescent girls were included if they were (1) enrolled in first year of secondary school and (2) not living in an institution or orphanage but within a family (as orphanages would have different characteristics than families). Girls were excluded if they (1) showed severe cognitive or psychiatric impairment that prohibited their ability to provide informed consent or comprehension of study requirements, (2) were unable or unwilling to complete the study, or (3) were not enrolled in school. Written informed consent from caregivers and assent from adolescents were obtained separately to prevent coercion.

Outcome Measures

We examined the impact of the intervention on 2 broad outcomes: (1) sexual risk-taking and (2) mental health among school-going adolescent girls. We evaluated study group differences in biomarker-based measures and self-reported sexual risk-taking behaviors and attitudes toward sexual risk-taking behaviors at postbaseline time points (i.e., 12 and 24 months).

Biomarker-based sexual risk. Adolescent girls who tested positive for HIV, gonorrhea, trichomoniasis, chlamydia, genital warts, or pregnancy were categorized as having a positive biomarker test for sexual risk-taking behavior (binary outcome). Because of the COVID-19 pandemic and the resulting school closures and social distancing requirements, study investigators adjusted the data collection protocol to minimize COVID-19 transmission. Hence, biomarker tests for HIV, STIs, and pregnancy were not conducted at 24 months but only at baseline and 12 months.

Self-reported sexual risk. Adolescent girls were asked the following questions:

1. Have you ever had sexual intercourse? (Yes or no)
2. The last time you had sexual intercourse (willingly or unwillingly), did you or your partner use a condom? (Yes or no)
3. Have you ever been diagnosed with any sexually transmitted disease (STDs)? (Yes or no) If yes, what disease? Chlamydia, herpes, trichomoniasis, syphilis, gonorrhea, genital warts, nonspecific disease, other (check all that apply).

If adolescent girls responded "yes" to "ever had sexual intercourse," indicated a diagnosis of STI, or did not use a condom during last sexual intercourse, they were categorized as engaging in sexual risk-taking based on self-reports (binary outcome).

Intentions and attitudes toward sexual risk-taking behaviors. We utilized 2 measures to assess intentions and

AJPH March 2023, Vol 113, No. 3

attitudes toward sexual risk-taking. The first measure, "sexual risk-taking intentions" was evaluated by a continuous summed score of 5 items (Cronbach $\alpha = 0.72$ at 12 and 24 months).[34] Participants were asked to rate their agreement with the following 5 statements:

1. I believe it's OK for people my age to have sex with someone they've just met.
2. I believe it's OK for people my age to have sex with someone they love.
3. I believe it's OK for people to have sex before marriage.
4. I agree it's OK to force a girlfriend/boyfriend to have sex even when they don't want to.
5. I believe it's OK to have sex without protection with someone you know.

Response options for each statement were never = 1; sometimes = 2; about half the time = 3; most of the time = 4; or always = 5. These 5 statements were summed and analyzed as a continuous variable, with higher scores indicative of greater agreement with sexual risk-taking.

The second measure assessed "Attitudes toward condom use" and comprised the following 3 items:

1. I think all people my age who have sex should use condoms.
2. Even if you know your partner very well you should use a condom.
3. I think it is very important to use condoms every time one has sex.

Response options were agree a great deal = 5; agree a lot = 4; moderately agree = 3; agree a little = 2; or not at all agree = 1. The 3 items had Cronbach $\alpha = 0.69$ (12 months) and 0.72 (24 months) and were summed and analyzed as a continuous score, with higher scores suggesting favorable attitudes toward condom use.

For mental health, we examined whether there were significant differences between groups only at 24 months after the intervention because findings on group differences at 12 months are reported in other papers published[35] and currently in press.[36] To get a comprehensive view of adolescents' overall mental well-being, we assessed 4 measures of mental health among adolescent girls: hopelessness, depressive symptoms, self-concept, and self-esteem. The psychological construct of hopelessness (whether girls have negative attitudes about the future) was measured using the 20-item Beck Hopelessness Scale (Cronbach $\alpha = 0.73$).[37] Girls were required to endorse pessimistic or deny optimistic statements. Hopelessness is common among depressed individuals and is associated with increased suicide risk.[39] Depressive symptoms were assessed using the 21-item Beck Depression Inventory (Cronbach $\alpha = 0.80$).[39] Depression is associated with sexual risk-taking behavior and other negative outcomes including suicidal ideation.[40] Self-concept (how girls think and feel about themselves) was evaluated using the 20-item Tennessee Self-Concept Scale (Cronbach $\alpha = 0.85$).[41] For this, girls self-reported ratings on their perception of identity and self-satisfaction. We used the 10-item Rosenberg Self-Esteem Scale to assess participants' self-esteem (Cronbach $\alpha = 0.71$).[42] This scale measures girls' self-worth by assessing both positive and negative feelings about the self. All items were reverse coded where required, and all items were summed and analyzed as continuous variables. Lower scores on the Beck Hopelessness Scale and the Beck Depressive Inventory are indicative of better mental health because these indicate less hopelessness and depressive symptoms. By contrast, higher scores on the Tennessee Self-Concept and Rosenberg Self-Esteem scales are better because these reflect higher levels of self-concept and self-esteem.

Statistical Analysis

All analyses were conducted in Stata version 17.0.[43] Characteristics of study participants at baseline are described in Table 1. We examined if there were any significant differences across study groups on baseline covariates listed in Table 1 (while adjusting for clustering by schools) and conducted sensitivity analyses to adjust for covariates that were significantly different across study groups.

We summarized the outcomes by study group and time point using means and standard deviations for continuous outcomes and numbers and percentages for categorical outcomes (Table 2). For continuous outcomes, we fitted 3-level mixed-effects models. Each model contained a fixed categorical effect for study group and time, the group-by-time interaction, and a random intercept at the school level. An unstructured residual-error covariance matrix of the residuals from the repeated assessments taken on the same participants was fitted, and the assumption of equal variances and covariances across groups was relaxed. For binary outcomes, each model contained fixed effects for study group and time, a group-by-time interaction term, and random intercepts at the school and participant levels, yielding a multilevel logistic regression model.

In both linear and logistic models, we estimated the variance–covariance matrices of parameter estimates by using robust Huber–White standard errors. We estimated the omnibus effects for

TABLE 1— Baseline Characteristics of Study Population: Suubi4her Study, Central Uganda, 2017–2022

Characteristics	Total (n = 1260), Mean ±SD or No. (%)	Usual Care (n = 408), Mean ±SD or No. (%)	YDA (n = 471), Mean ±SD or No. (%)	YDA+MFG (n = 381), Mean ±SD or No. (%)
Age, y	15.4 ±0.9	15.2 ±0.9	15.5 ±0.8	15.4 ±0.9
Orphanhood status[a]				
Double orphan	24 (1.9)	7 (1.7)	8 (1.7)	9 (2.4)
Single orphan	191 (15.2)	59 (14.5)	72 (15.3)	60 (15.8)
Nonorphan	1045 (82.9)	342 (83.8)	391 (83.0)	312 (81.9)
Primary caregiver				
Biological parents	965 (76.6)	312 (76.5)	370 (78.6)	283 (74.3)
Grandparents	140 (11.1)	46 (11.3)	54 (11.5)	40 (10.5)
Other relatives or nonrelatives	155 (12.3)	50 (12.2)	47 (10.0)	58 (15.2)
Primary caregiver employment status				
Formally employed	292 (23.2)	102 (25.0)	104 (22.1)	86 (22.6)
Not formally employed	968 (76.8)	306 (75.0)	367 (77.9)	295 (77.4)
Primary caregiver education level				
Did not go to school or completed all or part of primary-level education	496 (39.4)	144 (35.3)	186 (39.5)	166 (43.6)
Completed all or part of secondary-level education	319 (25.3)	115 (28.2)	110 (23.3)	94 (24.7)
Completed technical diploma or university degree	137 (10.9)	40 (9.8)	59 (12.5)	38 (10.0)
Don't know	308 (24.4)	109 (26.7)	116 (24.6)	83 (21.8)
Household size	7.0 ±2.7	6.8 ±2.6	7.0 ±2.7	7.2 ±2.9

Note. MFG = multiple family group; YDA = youth development account.
[a]Single orphan refers to 1 parent is still alive; double orphan refers to both parents are not alive.

study group, time, and the group-by-time interaction. We computed group-within-time effects regardless of the significance of the group-by-time interaction effect. To further elucidate time effects, we followed the statistically significant main effects for time with time-within-group simple effects comparisons. Because of the multiple pairwise comparisons, we performed adjustments to the *P* values using Sidak's method.

RESULTS

At baseline, 1260 school-going adolescent girls of mean age 15.4 years were enrolled. A total of 408 girls received usual care, 471 received YDA, and 381 received the combination intervention (YDA+MFG). There were no significant differences across study groups at baseline, except for participants' age ($P = .031$) with YDA group 0.31 years older than controls and no difference between other groups. Overall, most girls were nonorphans (82.9%) and being cared for by biological parents (76.6%; Table 1). Approximately 77% of primary caregivers were not formally employed, and approximately 11% completed a technical diploma or university degree. On average, girls resided in households with 7 people. At baseline, 7.3% (n = 92) of adolescent girls had a positive biological test for HIV, STIs, or pregnancy (Appendix, Table B). The most common STI diagnosis was for trichomoniasis (5.2%; n = 65). While only 8 girls (0.6%) were positive for HIV at baseline, 14 (1.1%) had a positive pregnancy test. At 24 months, the retention rate was 92.4%. The distribution of sexual risk-taking outcomes by study group and time point are presented in Table 2 and in the Appendix, Tables B and C.

Sexual Risk-Taking Behavior and Attitudes

For biomarker-based sexual risk, self-reported sexual risk, sexual risk-taking intentions, and attitudes toward condom use outcomes, we observed no significant differences between study groups at 12 and 24 months (Table 3).

Effects on Mental Health

There were significant group-by-time interaction effects for all mental health

TABLE 2— Summary of Sexual Risk-Taking and Mental Health Outcomes by Study Group and Timepoint: Suubi4her Study, Central Uganda, 2017–2022

Outcome	Study Arm	Baseline		12 mo		24 mo	
		No.	No. (%) or Mean ±SD	No.	No. (%) or Mean ±SD	No.	No. (%) or Mean ±SD
Sexual risk-taking							
Biomarker-based sexual risk	Control	408	29 (7.1)	396	15 (3.7)	NA	NA
	YDA	471	43 (9.1)	457	22 (4.7)	NA	NA
	YDA+MFG	381	20 (5.3)	366	22 (5.8)	NA	NA
	Entire sample	1260	92 (7.3)	1219	59 (4.8)	NA	NA
Self-reported sexual risk	Control	408	23 (5.6)	396	34 (8.6)	380	44 (10.8)
	YDA	471	15 (3.2)	457	52 (11.4)	441	75 (15.9)
	YDA+MFG	381	19 (5.0)	366	29 (7.9)	344	55 (14.4)
	Entire sample	1260	57 (4.5)	1219	115 (9.4)	1165	174 (14.9)
Sexual risk-taking intentions (5-item scale)	Control	408	7.5 ±3.9	396	8.5 ±4.0	380	7.9 ±3.7
	YDA	471	7.5 ±3.6	457	8.6 ±4.3	441	7.7 ±3.4
	YDA+MFG	381	7.5 ±3.8	366	8.2 ±4.1	344	7.8 ±3.6
	Entire sample	1260	7.5 ±3.7	1219	8.5 ±4.1	1165	7.8 ±3.5
Attitudes toward condom use (3-item scale)	Control	408	10.4 ±4.4	396	11.3 ±3.6	380	12.0 ±3.5
	YDA	471	10.9 ±4.3	457	11.2 ±3.7	441	11.8 ±3.7
	YDA+MFG	381	11.1 ±4.2	366	11.0 ±3.7	344	11.9 ±3.6
	Entire sample	1260	10.8 ±4.3	1219	11.2 ±3.7	1165	11.9 ±3.6
Mental health							
Hopelessness	Control	408	4.9 ±2.8	396	4.4 ±2.7	380	4.7 ±2.9
	YDA	471	5.0 ±2.8	457	4.0 ±2.5	441	4.2 ±2.7
	YDA+MFG	381	5.1 ±2.9	366	4.0 ±2.5	344	4.0 ±2.5
	Entire sample	1260	5.0 ±2.9	1219	4.1 ±2.5	1165	4.2 ±2.5
Depression	Control	408	19.2 ±10.3	396	16.6 ±9.8	380	14.8 ±9.3
	YDA	471	17.8 ±10.2	457	14.3 ±8.8	441	13.5 ±8.6
	YDA+MFG	381	18.5 ±10.1	366	13.8 ±9.1	344	12.0 ±8.8
	Entire sample	1260	18.5 ±10.2	1219	14.8 ±9.1	1165	13.5 ±8.8
Self-concept	Control	408	80.6 ±11.5	379	81.9 ±12.0	347	81.3 ±12.4
	YDA	471	81.1 ±11.8	408	84.4 ±10.5	377	83.3 ±11.8
	YDA+MFG	381	80.7 ±12.7	335	84.0 ±10.5	303	84.4 ±11.5
	Entire sample	1260	80.8 ±12.0	1122	83.4 ±11.1	1027	82.4 ±11.5
Self-esteem	Control	408	32.9 ±5.6	396	33.0 ±5.7	380	35.8 ±4.4
	YDA	471	33.3 ±5.6	457	34.5 ±4.5	441	36.2 ±3.9
	YDA+MFG	380	32.7 ±5.4	366	34.6 ±4.2	344	36.4 ±3.9
	Entire sample	1259	33.0 ±5.4	1219	34.0 ±4.9	1165	36.4 ±3.9

Note. MFG = multiple family group; NA = not applicable (biological tests for HIV and other sexually transmitted infections were not conducted at 24-month follow-up because of study protocol adjustments made to reduce the spread of COVID-19); YDA = youth development account.

outcomes (Appendix, Table D). At 24 months, we observed adolescent girls in both YDA and YDA+MFG intervention groups had significantly lower levels of depressive symptoms and significantly better self-concept than controls. For hopelessness, only girls in the combination intervention arm (YDA+MFG) had significantly lower levels of hopelessness than controls (Table 4). However, there were no study group differences for self-esteem. For all the sexual risk-taking and mental health outcomes, there were no significant differences between the YDA and

TABLE 3— Study Group Differences of Predicted Probabilities and Estimated Mean Differences Within Each Time Point for Sexual Risk-Taking Behavior: Suubi4her Study, Central Uganda, 2017–2022

Timepoint	Group Comparison	Biomarker-Based Sexual Risk, RD (95% CI)	Self-Reported Sexual Risk, RD (95% CI)	Sexual Risk-Taking Intentions, EMD (95% CI)	Attitudes Toward Condom Use, EMD (95% CI)
12 mo	YDA vs control	0.01 (−0.07, 0.10)	0.02 (−0.04, 0.09)	0.09 (−0.47, 0.66)	−0.13 (−1.28, 1.01)
	YDA+MFG vs control	−0.01 (−0.08, 0.04)	−0.01 (−0.06, 0.04)	−0.36 (−1.03, 0.33)	−0.36 (−1.36, 0.64)
	YDA+MFG vs YDA	−0.03 (−0.11, 0.04)	−0.03 (−0.10, 0.03)	−0.44 (−1.08, 0.19)	−0.22 (−0.98, 0.53)
24 mo	YDA vs control	NA	0.05 (−0.01, 0.11)	−0.17 (−0.86, 0.50)	−0.36 (−0.98, 0.26)
	YDA+MFG vs control	NA	0.04 (−0.01, 0.08)	−0.18 (−1.32, 0.96)	−0.13 (−0.77, 0.50)
	YDA+MFG vs YDA	NA	−0.01 (−0.08, 0.52)	−0.00 (−1.03, 1.01)	0.23 (−0.41, 0.87)
No. of participants		1260	1260	1260	2260
No. of observations		2520	3780	3644	3644

Note. CI = confidence interval; EMD = differences of estimated marginal means; MFG = multiple family group; NA = not applicable (biological tests for HIV and sexually transmitted infections were not conducted at 24-month follow-up because of study protocol adjustments made to reduce the spread of COVID-19); RD = differences of predicted probabilities; YDA = youth development account. Group-within-time simple effects.

YDA+MFG intervention groups. Simple effects comparing follow-ups to baseline within the significant time main effect appear in the Appendix, Table E.

Sensitivity analysis results were substantively unchanged after we adjusted for age (Appendix, Tables F–I).

DISCUSSION

School-going adolescent girls in SSA require special attention to reduce their vulnerability to HIV infection and poor mental health. Economic empowerment and family strengthening interventions can play an important role in improving financial resources[44,45] while equipping families to deal with the stressors of living in poverty-impacted environments.[46] In this population of secondary school–going adolescent girls, we observed no significant differences between study groups at postbaseline time points for objective biomarker-based and self-reported sexual risk-taking behaviors and attitudes. This finding aligns with a previous study among adolescents living with HIV in which no differences in sexual risk-taking attitudes were observed between the intervention and control group.[34]

Research conducted among adolescents in the Rakai district of Uganda over a 17-year period consistently showed the highest prevalence of sexual experience was among adolescents aged 19 years and the lowest among adolescents aged 15 years.[47] The prevalence was significantly lower among adolescents enrolled in school versus adolescents out of school across all ages. Hence, the lack of significant findings could be attributable to the young age of participants and because all participants were in school and residing within families. Given these reasons, it is not surprising only a small proportion

TABLE 4— Study Group Differences of Estimated Marginal Means Within Each Time Point for Mental Health Outcomes: Suubi4her Study, Central Uganda, 2017–2022

Timepoint	Group Comparison	Hopelessness, EMD (95% CI)	Depression, EMD (95% CI)	Self-Concept, EMD (95% CI)	Self-Esteem, EMD (95% CI)
24 mo	YDA vs control	−0.29 (−0.71, 0.12)	−1.38 (−2.63, −0.12)	1.96 (0.07, 3.85)	0.34 (−0.24, 0.92)
	YDA+MFG vs control	−0.45 (−0.90, −0.01)	−2.80 (−4.29, −1.32)	3.04 (0.95, 5.12)	0.53 (−0.12, 1.19)
	YDA+MFG vs YDA	−0.15 (−0.54, 0.23)	−1.42 (−2.95, 0.11)	1.08 (−0.90, 3.05)	0.19 (−0.36, 0.75)
No. of participants		1260	1260	1260	1260
No. of observations		3644	3644	3409	3643

Note. CI = confidence interval; EMD = differences of estimated marginal means; MFG = multiple family group; YDA = youth development account. Group-within-time simple effects.

of adolescent girls had a positive self-report of engaging in sexual risk-taking behavior (4.5% at baseline, 9.4% at 12 months, and 14.9% at 24 months) or had a positive biomarker test for HIV, other STIs, or pregnancy (7.3% at baseline and 4.8% at 12 months). Furthermore, only 3.3% were sexually active at baseline and, as expected, this increased to 9.4% at 24 months.

Similarly, for sexual risk-taking intentions and attitudes toward condom use, we observed no significant differences by study group. However, for girls in the YDA group, our time-within-group analyses located a slight increase in sexual risk-taking intentions at 12 months but more favorable attitudes to condom use at 24 months compared with baseline. Girls in the YDA+MFG group had more favorable attitudes toward condom use at 24 months compared with baseline (Appendix, Table E). This highlights the urgent need for better refined sexual risk-reduction interventions for adolescent girls in the transition period. Over time, the YDA and family strengthening activities appeared to improve attitudes toward condom use, although sexual risk-taking intentions appear to have increased.

At 24-month follow-up, we observed differential effects by study group for all mental health outcomes except self-esteem. The YDA and YDA+MFG interventions were more efficacious in reducing girls' depressive symptoms and improving self-concept than usual care. This meant that both YDA and YDA+MFG interventions had sustained effects on reducing depressive symptoms and improving self-concept among adolescent girls at 24 months. Moreover, only the YDA+MFG intervention was effective in reducing feelings of hopelessness among girls compared with usual care at 24 months. These are important findings that reinforce the need for economic empowerment interventions that improve families' financial resources as important for improving adolescents' mental health.

Our findings align with previous studies that found economic empowerment interventions positively improved mental health of vulnerable populations in SSA.[44] They also speak to the wide applicability and effectiveness of MFG interventions. Previous studies observed the beneficial impact of MFG interventions on reducing depressive symptoms, improving self-concept, and reducing oppositional defiant disorder and impaired functioning among children with disruptive behavior disorders in Uganda.[45] Similarly, MFG interventions have been adapted and implemented among youth living with HIV in the United States and South Africa, with positive results.[48,49] The open communication, shared experiences, and social support networks built during Suubi4-Her MFG sessions are likely to have contributed to better mental health even among adolescent girls. Given that MFG is sensitive to cultural norms and tailored to the local environment, incorporating MFG components into future interventions designed to prevent sexual risk-taking and prevent poor mental health may have tremendous potential.

Limitations

Despite numerous strengths in the study design, there were a few limitations worth highlighting. First, self-reported findings (specifically, self-reported sexual risk and intentions and attitudes toward sexual risk-taking behaviors) may be subject to underreporting with adolescents providing socially desirable responses. Sexual behavior and mental health are topics that are heavily stigmatized in conservative African communities.[50,51] Although we did conduct biological tests for other STIs, this was done once per year, and so it is likely that we could have missed some infection windows if participants became infected and then received STI treatment and the illness resolved between the assessment intervals—although STI treatment among poor school-going adolescents like the ones included in the study is rare.

Second, our findings are not generalizable to out-of-school adolescent girls, at the time of study recruitment, who may be at higher risk of sexual risk-taking and poor mental health. Third, this analysis was done on the entire sample of all adolescent girls, including investigating sexual risk-taking intentions among those who were not sexually active. Analyses may show different trends and a different impact of the intervention on sexual risk-taking attitudes and behaviors if the sample comprised only girls who were sexually active.

Conclusions

On one hand, we found that providing YDA in addition to family strengthening activities to adolescent girls in secondary schools in poverty-impacted communities in Uganda has the potential to positively improve their mental health. However, our analyses show no significant differences across groups on sexual risk-taking behaviors, something that could be explained by the relatively young age of the participants enrolled in the study. Future studies may consider replicating these interventions and analyses in an older population of adolescent girls, including those transitioning into young adults who are likely to be more sexually active. AJPH

ABOUT THE AUTHORS

Fred M. Ssewamala and Rachel Brathwaite are with the International Center for Child Health and Development, Brown School, Washington University in St Louis, MO. Torsten B. Neilands is with the Division of Prevention Science, University of California, San Francisco.

CORRESPONDENCE

Correspondence should be sent to Fred M. Ssewamala, William E. Gordon Distinguished Professor, Brown School, Washington University in St Louis, St Louis, MO 63130 (e-mail: fms1@wustl.edu). Reprints can be ordered at https://ajph.org by clicking the "Reprints" link.

PUBLICATION INFORMATION

Full Citation: Ssewamala FM, Brathwaite R, Neilands TB. Economic empowerment, HIV risk behavior, and mental health among school-going adolescent girls in Uganda: longitudinal cluster-randomized controlled trial, 2017–2022. *Am J Public Health*. 2023;113(3):306–315.

Acceptance Date: November 3, 2022.

DOI: https://doi.org/10.2105/AJPH.2022.307169

CONTRIBUTORS

F. M. Ssewamala conceptualized and designed the Suubi4Her Study on which this article is based, acquired funding for the Suubi4Her study, supervised the work, and reviewed and edited the article. R. Brathwaite performed the data analysis and wrote the initial draft of the article. T. B. Neilands provided statistical guidance on the analysis and reviewed and edited the article. All authors provided critical inputs and edits to the article and its revisions and approved the final article for submission.

ACKNOWLEDGMENTS

The study outlined in this protocol is supported by the National Institute of Mental Health (NIMH) under award 1R01MH113486-01 (PI: Fred M. Ssewamala, PhD).

We are grateful to Abel Mwebembezi at Reach the Youth–Uganda, Joseph Kato Bakulu at Masaka Catholic Diocese, Gertrude Nakigozi and Godfrey Kigozi at Rakai Health Sciences Program in Uganda, and Phionah Namatovu and Sarah Namutebi at the International Center for Child Health and Development for their respective contributions to the study design and implementation. In addition, we are grateful to the financial institutions that agreed to work with the adolescent girls in opening savings accounts and the extension workers who have committed time to train the adolescent girls in conducting income-generating activities. Our thanks also go to the Ugandan Government Ministry of Education and the 47 secondary schools that have agreed to participate in the Suubi4Her study.

Note. The content is solely the responsibility of the authors and does not necessarily represent the official views of NIMH or the National Institutes of Health.

CONFLICTS OF INTEREST

The authors declare no conflicts of interest.

HUMAN PARTICIPANT PROTECTION

The Suubi4Her study was conducted in accordance with the Declaration of Helsinki and approved by the Washington University in St Louis institutional review board (IRB no. 201703102), the Uganda Virus Research Institute (GC/127/17/07/619), and the Uganda National Council of Science and Technology (SS4406). The study is also registered in the ClinicalTrials.gov database (Identifier: NCT03307226).

REFERENCES

1. UNICEF. Adolescent HIV prevention: HIV in adolescents. 2020. Available at: https://data.unicef.org/topic/hivaids/adolescents-young-people. Accessed June 22, 2021.
2. UNICEF. Turning the tide against AIDS will require more concentrated focus on adolescents and young people. UNICEF Data. 2017. Available at: https://data.unicef.org/topic/hiv-aids. Accessed April 28, 2022.
3. Cortina MA, Sodha A, Fazel M, Ramchandani PG. Prevalence of child mental health problems in sub-Saharan Africa: a systematic review. *Arch Pediatr Adolesc Med*. 2012;166(3):276–281. https://doi.org/10.1001/archpediatrics.2011.592
4. Campbell OLK, Bann D, Patalay P. The gender gap in adolescent mental health: a cross-national investigation of 566,829 adolescents across 73 countries. *SSM Popul Health*. 2021;13:100742. https://doi.org/10.1016/j.ssmph.2021.100742
5. Abbo C, Kinyanda E, Kizza RB, Levin J, Ndyanabangi S, Stein DJ. Prevalence, comorbidity and predictors of anxiety disorders in children and adolescents in rural north-eastern Uganda. *Child Adolesc Psychiatry Ment Health*. 2013;7(1):21. https://doi.org/10.1186/1753-2000-7-21
6. Rescorla L, Achenbach T, Ivanova MY, et al. Behavioral and emotional problems reported by parents of children ages 6 to 16 in 31 societies. *J Emot Behav Disord*. 2007;15(3):130–142. https://doi.org/10.1177/10634266070150030101
7. Glynn JR, Caraël M, Auvert B, et al. Why do young women have a much higher prevalence of HIV than young men? A study in Kisumu, Kenya and Ndola, Zambia. *AIDS*. 2001;15(suppl 4):S51–S60. https://doi.org/10.1097/00002030-200108004-00006
8. Barhafumwa B, Dietrich J, Closson K, et al. High prevalence of depression symptomology among adolescents in Soweto, South Africa associated with being female and cofactors relating to HIV transmission. *Vulnerable Child Youth Stud*. 2016;11(3):263–273. https://doi.org/10.1080/17450128.2016.1198854
9. UNAIDS. Women and HIV. A spotlight on adolescent girls and young women. 2019. Available at: https://www.unaids.org/sites/default/files/media_asset/2019_women-and-hiv_en.pdf. Accessed April 29, 2022.
10. UNICEF Uganda Country Office. Multidimensional child poverty and deprivation in Uganda: Volume 1. 2019. Available at: https://www.unicef.org/uganda/reports/multidimensional-child-poverty-and-deprivation-uganda-report-volume-1. Accessed May 1, 2022.
11. African Development Bank Group. *Uganda Country Gender Profile*. February 2016. Available at: https://www.afdb.org/fileadmin/uploads/afdb/Documents/Project-and-Operations/UGANDA_COUNTRY_GENDER_PROFILE-2016.pdf. Accessed May 4, 2022.
12. African Development Bank Group. HIV & AIDS and supportive learning environments. Good policy and practice in HIV & AIDS in education (booklet series). Paris, France: UNESCO; 2008.
13. Pettifor AE, Levandowski BA, MacPhail C, Padian NS, Cohen MS, Rees HV. Keep them in school: the importance of education as a protective factor against HIV infection among young South African women. *Int J Epidemiol*. 2008;37(6):1266–1273. https://doi.org/10.1093/ije/dyn131
14. Nobelius A-M, Kalina B, Pool R, Whitworth J, Chesters J, Power R. Sexual partner types and related sexual health risk among out-of-school adolescents in rural south-west Uganda. *AIDS Care*. 2011;23(2):252–259. https://doi.org/10.1080/09540121.2010.507736
15. Green C, Mukuria A, Rubin D. Addressing early marriage in Uganda. Washington, DC: USAID, Futures Group, Health Policy Initiative, Task Order I; 2009.
16. Kigozi F, Ssebunnya J, Kizza D, Cooper S, Ndyanabangi S. An overview of Uganda's mental health care system: results from an assessment using the World Health Organization's Assessment Instrument for Mental Health Systems (WHO-AIMS). *Int J Ment Health Syst*. 2010;4(1):1–9. https://doi.org/10.1186/1752-4458-4-1
17. Cooper K, Stewart K. Does money affect children's outcomes? A systematic review. Joseph Rowntree Foundation. 2013. Available at: https://www.jrf.org.uk/sites/default/files/jrf/migrated/files/money-children-outcomes-full.pdf. Accessed May 2, 2022.
18. Cooper K, Stewart K. Does money affect children's outcomes? An update. Centre for Analysis of Social Exclusion. 2017. Available at: https://sticerd.lse.ac.uk/dps/case/cp/casepaper203.pdf. Accessed May 2, 2022.
19. Whiteford HA, Degenhardt L, Rehm J, et al. Global burden of disease attributable to mental and substance use disorders: findings from the Global Burden of Disease Study 2010. *Lancet*. 2013;382(9904):1575–1586. https://doi.org/10.1016/S0140-6736(13)61611-6
20. O'Donnell L, O'Donnell CR, Stueve A. Early sexual initiation and subsequent sex-related risks among urban minority youth: the Reach for Health Study. *Fam Plann Perspect*. 2001;33(6):268–275. https://doi.org/10.2307/3030194
21. Brookmeyer KA, Henrich CC. Disentangling adolescent pathways of sexual risk taking. *J Prim Prev*. 2009;30(6):677–696. https://doi.org/10.1007/s10935-009-0196-6
22. Armistead L, Kotchick B, Forehand R. Teenage pregnancy, sexually transmitted diseases, and HIV/AIDS. *Handbook of Preventive Interventions for Children and Adolescents*. Hoboken, NJ: John Wiley and Sons; 2004:227–254.

23. Remien RH, Stirratt MJ, Nguyen N, Robbins RN, Pala AN, Mellins CA. Mental health and HIV/AIDS: the need for an integrated response. *AIDS.* 2019; 33(9):1411–1420. https://doi.org/10.1097/QAD.0000000000002227

24. Patel V, Araya R, Chatterjee S, et al. Treatment and prevention of mental disorders in low-income and middle-income countries. *Lancet.* 2007;370(9591):991–1005. https://doi.org/10.1016/S0140-6736(07)61240-9

25. Ssewamala FM, Bermudez LG, Neilands TB, et al. Suubi4Her: a study protocol to examine the impact and cost associated with a combination intervention to prevent HIV risk behavior and improve mental health functioning among adolescent girls in Uganda. *BMC Public Health.* 2018;18(1):693. https://doi.org/10.1186/s12889-018-5604-5

26. Sherraden M. *Assets and the Poor: A New American Welfare Policy.* New York, NY: ME Sharpe; 1991:344.

27. Sherraden M. Stakeholding: notes on a theory of welfare based on assets. *Soc Serv Rev.* 1990; 64(4):580–601. https://doi.org/10.1086/603797

28. Ghandour RM, Kogan MD, Blumberg SJ, Jones JR, Perrin JM. Mental health conditions among school-aged children: geographic and sociodemographic patterns in prevalence and treatment. *J Dev Behav Pediatr.* 2012;33(1):42–54. https://doi.org/10.1097/DBP.0b013e31823e18fd

29. McKay MM, Gonzales JJ, Stone S, Ryland D, Kohner K. Multiple family therapy groups. *Soc Work Groups.* 1995;18(4):41–56. https://doi.org/10.1300/J009v18n04_04

30. McNeely C, Shew ML, Beuhring T, Sieving R, Miller BC, Blum RWM. Mothers' influence on the timing of first sex among 14- and 15-year-olds. *J Adolesc Health.* 2002;31(3):256–265. https://doi.org/10.1016/S1054-139X(02)00350-6

31. Askelson NM, Campo S, Smith S. Mother–daughter communication about sex: the influence of authoritative parenting style. *Health Commun.* 2012;27(5):439–448. https://doi.org/10.1080/10410236.2011.606526

32. Widman L, Choukas-Bradley S, Noar SM, Nesi J, Garrett K. Parent–adolescent sexual communication and adolescent safer sex behavior: a meta-analysis. *JAMA Pediatr.* 2016;170(1):52–61. https://doi.org/10.1001/jamapediatrics.2015.2731

33. The Republic of Uganda. The HIV and AIDS Uganda country progress report 2014. June 15, 2015. Available at: http://www.unaids.org/sites/default/files/country/documents/UGA_narrative_report_2015.pdf. Accessed September 26, 2022.

34. Shato T, Nabunya P, Byansi W, et al. Family economic empowerment, family social support, and sexual risk-taking behaviors among adolescents living with HIV in Uganda: the Suubi+Adherence Study. *J Adolesc Health.* 2021;69(3):406–413. https://doi.org/10.1016/j.jadohealth.2021.02.005

35. Byansi W, Ssewamala FM, Neilands TB, et al. The short-term impact of a combination intervention on depressive symptoms among school-going adolescent girls in southwestern Uganda: the Suubi4Her cluster randomized trial. *J Adolesc Health.* 2022;71(3):301–307. https://doi.org/10.1016/j.jadohealth.2022.04.008

36. Filiatreau LM, Tutlam NT, Brathwaite R, et al. Effects of a combination economic empowerment and family strengthening intervention on psychosocial well-being among Ugandan adolescent girls and young women: analysis of a cluster randomized controlled trial from the Suubi4Her study. *J Adolesc Health.* In press.

37. Beck AT, Weissman A, Lester D, Trexler L. The measurement of pessimism: the hopelessness scale. *J Consult Clin Psychol.* 1974;42(6):861–865. https://doi.org/10.1037/h0037562

38. Brown GK, Beck AT, Steer RA, Grisham JR. Risk factors for suicide in psychiatric outpatients: a 20-year prospective study. *J Consult Clin Psychol.* 2000;68(3):371–377. https://doi.org/10.1037/0022-006X.68.3.371

39. Beck AT, Ward CH, Mendelson M, Mock J, Erbaugh J. An inventory for measuring depression. *Arch Gen Psychiatry.* 1961;4(6):561–571. https://doi.org/10.1001/archpsyc.1961.01710120031004

40. Uddin R, Burton NW, Maple M, Khan SR, Khan A. Suicidal ideation, suicide planning, and suicide attempts among adolescents in 59 low-income and middle-income countries: a population-based study. *Lancet Child Adolesc Health.* 2019; 3(4):223–233. https://doi.org/10.1016/S2352-4642(18)30403-6

41. Fitts WH, Warren WL. *Tennessee Self-Concept Scale, TSCS 2. Manual.* 2nd ed. Los Angeles, CA: Western Psychological Services; 1997.

42. Rosenberg M. The measurement of self-esteem. In: *Society and the Adolescent Self-Image.* Princeton, NJ: Princeton University Press; 1965. https://doi.org/10.1515/9781400876136

43. Stata Statistical Software: Release 17. College Station, TX: StataCorp LLC; 2021.

44. Ssewamala FM, Shu-Huah Wang J, Brathwaite R, et al. Impact of a family economic intervention (Bridges) on health functioning of adolescents orphaned by HIV/AIDS: a 5-year (2012–2017) cluster randomized controlled trial in Uganda. *Am J Public Health.* 2021;111(3):504–513. https://doi.org/10.2105/AJPH.2020.306044

45. Brathwaite R, Ssewamala FM, Mutumba M, et al. The long-term (5-year) impact of a family economic empowerment intervention on adolescents living with HIV in Uganda: analysis of longitudinal data from a cluster randomized controlled trial from the Suubi+Adherence Study (2012–2018). *AIDS Behav.* 2022;26(10):3337–3344. https://doi.org/10.1007/s10461-022-03637-1

46. Brathwaite R, Ssewamala FM, Sensoy Bahar O, et al. The longitudinal impact of an evidence-based multiple family group intervention (Amaka Amasanyufu) on oppositional defiant disorder and impaired functioning among children in Uganda: analysis of a cluster randomized trial from the SMART Africa-Uganda scale-up study (2016–2022). *J Child Psychol Psychiatry.* 2022; 63(11):1252–1260. https://doi.org/10.1111/jcpp.13566

47. Santelli JS, Song X, Holden IK, et al. Prevalence of sexual experience and initiation of sexual intercourse among adolescents, Rakai District, Uganda, 1994–2011. *J Adolesc Health.* 2015;57(5): 496–505. https://doi.org/10.1016/j.jadohealth.2015.07.018

48. McKay MM, Chasse KT, Paikoff R, et al. Family-level impact of the CHAMP Family Program: a community collaborative effort to support urban families and reduce youth HIV risk exposure. *Fam Process.* 2004;43(1):79–93. https://doi.org/10.1111/j.1545-5300.2004.04301007.x

49. Mellins CA, Nestadt D, Bhana A, et al. Adapting evidence-based interventions to meet the needs of adolescents growing up with HIV in South Africa: the VUKA case example. *Glob Soc Welf.* 2014;1(3):97–110. https://doi.org/10.1007/s40609-014-0023-8

50. Abdallah AK, Magata RJ, Sylvester JN. Barriers to parent–child communication on sexual and reproductive health issues in East Africa: a review of qualitative research in four countries. *J Afr Stud Dev.* 2017;9(4):45–50. https://doi.org/10.5897/JASD2016.0410

51. Ssebunnya J, Kigozi F, Lund C, Kizza D, Okello E. Stakeholder perceptions of mental health stigma and poverty in Uganda. *BMC Int Health Hum Rights.* 2009;9(1):5. https://doi.org/10.1186/1472-698X-9-5

Use of Judicial Bypass of Mandatory Parental Consent to Access Abortion and Judicial Bypass Denials, Florida and Texas, 2018–2021

Amanda Jean Stevenson, PhD, and Kate Coleman-Minahan, RN, PhD, FNP-BC

AJPH March 2023, Vol 113, No. 3

Objectives. To describe minors' use of judicial bypass to access abortion and the percentage of bypass petitions denied in Florida and Texas.

Methods. Data were derived from official state statistics on judicial bypasses and abortions by age in Texas and Florida; abortions in Texas among minor nonresidents were estimated. In addition, judicial bypass petitions as a percentage of abortions received by minors and judicial bypass denials as a percentage of petitions were calculated.

Results. Between 2018 and 2021, minors received 5527 abortions in Florida and an estimated 5220 abortions in Texas. Use of judicial bypass was stable at 14% to 15% in Florida and declined from 14% to 10% in Texas. Among petitions for judicial bypass, denials increased in Florida from 6% to a maximum of 13% and remained stable in Texas at 5% to 7%.

Conclusions. Minors' use of judicial bypass in Texas and Florida is substantial. The percentage of denials is higher and increasing in Florida.

Public Health Implications. Minors who need confidential abortion care may now be forced to seek judicial bypass far from home. Parental involvement laws in states that do not ban abortion will compound barriers to abortion care. (*Am J Public Health*. 2023;113(3):316–319. https://doi.org/10.2105/AJPH.2022.307173)

State-level abortion bans have expanded since the Supreme Court ended constitutional protection of abortion care in June 2022. For residents of states that ban abortion care, traveling to another state to obtain care may still be complicated by restrictive abortion laws in the state where care is sought. Here we call attention to one type of restriction, state parental involvement laws, which mandate that minors notify or secure consent from one or both parents before receiving abortion care unless they petition a judge for bypass of parental involvement.

For minors forced out of state, parental involvement laws will increase barriers to receiving timely abortion care. Once a state bans abortion, minors who would have sought bypasses there will need both care and bypasses out of state if they travel to a state with parental involvement laws.

Currently, 22 states that have not banned abortion still enforce parental involvement laws. Previous work demonstrates that parental involvement laws do not increase parental support[1] and jeopardize adolescents' health and well-being by restricting and delaying care,[2,3] increasing the likelihood of abuse from parents[4,5] and sometimes forcing them to seek judicial bypass.

Obtaining judicial bypass involves overcoming numerous logistical hurdles[3,6,7] to request a bypass of parental involvement in an often humiliating and sometimes traumatizing court hearing.[6] Navigating and enduring this process far from home could prove an insurmountable barrier.

Texas and Florida are the 2 most populous states that enforce parental consent; Florida moved from parental notification to consent in 2020. Texas is now enforcing a total abortion ban.[8] Florida may follow soon, but until it does the state is regionally consequential for abortion access and the rate of denials is salient as adolescents choose where to travel for care.

The fraction of minors who use judicial bypass to access abortion and how often judges deny bypass petitions are not systematically reported. To generate evidence needed to develop clinical, legal, and practical support for adolescents in states that mandate parental involvement, we calculated annual numbers of bypass petitions, estimated annual percentages of abortions obtained by minor adolescents after bypass, and annual percentages of bypass petitions denied by judges in Texas and Florida between 2018 and 2021.

METHODS

Data on number of judicial bypass petitions filed, number of bypass petitions denied, and number of abortions provided to minors were obtained for Texas and Florida annually between 2018 and 2021. Annual counts of judicial bypass petitions filed and denied during that period were obtained by request from the Florida Office of State Courts Administration and from the Web site of the Texas Office of Court Administration.[9]

Because minors are subject to parental involvement laws in the state where they receive care, the best measure of the population potentially needing a judicial bypass of parental consent is abortion incidence among people younger than 18 years, including residents and nonresidents. Data on annual numbers of abortions obtained by minors in Florida were requested from the Florida Agency for Health Care Administration for 2018 to 2021. Annual numbers of Texas resident abortions among minors are publicly available for 2018 to 2021, but nonresident Texas abortions are reported by age group, with 1 age group (15–19 years) comprising both minors and nonminors. Therefore, we estimated annual abortions in Texas for nonresident minors. Estimation procedures are described in the Appendix (available as a supplement to the online version of this article at http://www.ajph.org). For each state and year, we computed bypass petitions as a percentage of abortions among minors and bypass petitions denied as a percentage of all bypasses.

RESULTS

Between 2018 and 2021, judicial bypass as a percentage of minors who obtained abortions in Florida was stable at 14% to 15% (from 193 petitions per 1398 abortions to 216 per 1406). In Texas, use of judicial bypass declined over the study period from 14% to 10% (from 205 per 1437 to 107 per 1081; Figure 1).

Denials of judicial bypasses increased in Florida from 6% to 9% between 2018 and 2019. In 2020, when Florida's parental involvement law changed from notification to consent, denials of judicial bypass rose to 13% before declining slightly to 12% the next year. In Texas, the percentage of judicial bypasses denied remained relatively flat, ranging from 5% to 7% over the study period.

DISCUSSION

In this study, we found that substantial numbers of adolescents rely on judicial bypass and that bypasses are routinely denied in both Florida and Texas. About 15% of minors obtaining abortion care in Florida used judicial bypass annually between 2018 and 2021. In Texas, this percentage declined from 14% to 10% during the study period, a trend that may be due to the increasing barriers to abortion in the state, which likely impact the most marginalized groups.[8]

Over our study period, denials as a percentage of judicial bypass petitions doubled in Florida. This increase was most marked after 2020, when Florida's law changed from parental notification to consent, a pattern also observed after Texas made its bypass process more burdensome in 2016.[2] Texas has coordinated support for bypass seekers, whereas Florida does not, which could partly explain the higher level of denials in Florida later in the period and the steady rate of denials in Texas. Coordinated support networks are poised to become even more important in states maintaining abortion access.

Reasons for denials are not released, but previous research has shown that some Texas judges deny bypasses on grounds not supported by law, such as gestational duration or family socioeconomic status.[6,10]

Here we have described 2 basic statistics researchers and public health practitioners should construct as part of monitoring the effects of forced parental involvement laws: the extent of minors' reliance on judicial bypass to access abortion care (measured as bypasses as a percentage of abortions among minors) and the percentage of judicial bypasses denied.

Our study was limited by our inability to link judicial bypass petitions by petitioner. Individuals could have filed more than once and may not have received an abortion, resulting in overestimation of reliance on bypass to access abortion. In our estimates of nonresident Texas abortions, we assumed that the ratio of minor to nonminor Texas abortions was the same for residents and nonresidents,

AJPH March 2023, Vol 113, No. 3

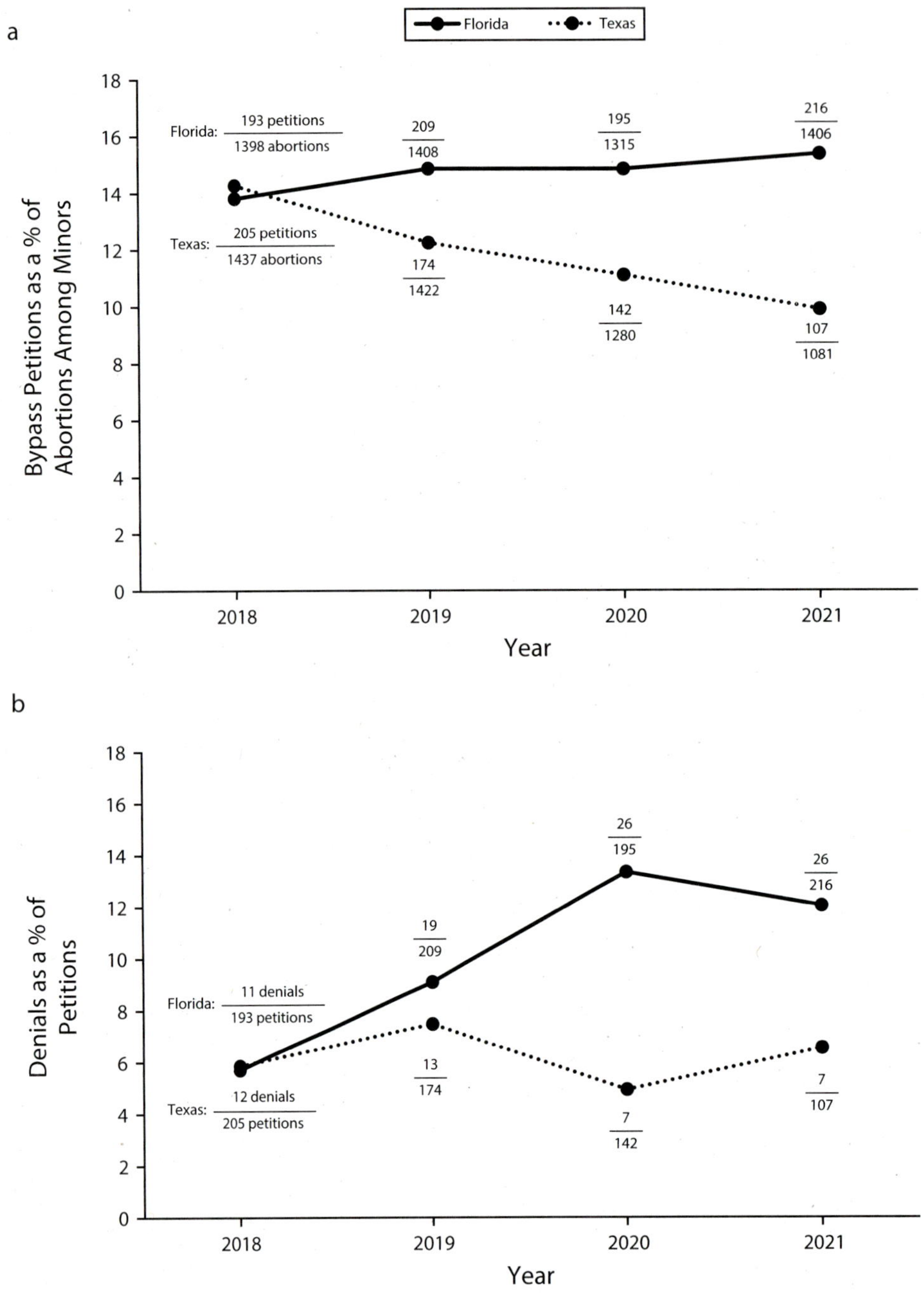

FIGURE 1— Judicial Bypass Petitions and Petition Denials in Florida and Texas: 2018–2021

which is conservative because it likely led us to overestimate denominators.

PUBLIC HEALTH IMPLICATIONS

By estimating the percentages of young people who rely on judicial bypass in states that totally ban or are expected to totally ban abortion, we have demonstrated that hundreds of minors who may be forced to travel for care could need judicial bypasses if their best option is a state with a parental involvement law. Minors from states that ban abortion must either strategically travel to states without parental involvement laws or face forced parental involvement or judicial bypass in a state that is not their home, further delaying care and possibly resulting in abortion denial. To develop clinical, legal, and practical support for minors, states that allow abortion access but mandate parental involvement, such as Colorado and Maryland, should routinely report the percentage of minors using judicial bypass and the percentage of denials as basic abortion surveillance data. AJPH

ABOUT THE AUTHORS

Amanda Jean Stevenson is with the Department of Sociology and the University of Colorado Population Center, University of Colorado, Boulder. Kate Coleman-Minahan is with the College of Nursing, University of Colorado Anschutz Medical Campus, and the University of Colorado Population Center, University of Colorado, Boulder.

CORRESPONDENCE

Correspondence should be sent to Amanda Jean Stevenson, PhD, Department of Sociology, UCB 327 Ketchum 195, Boulder, CO 80309 (e-mail: amanda.stevenson@colorado.edu). Reprints can be ordered at http://www.ajph.org by clicking the "Reprints" link.

PUBLICATION INFORMATION

Full Citation: Stevenson AJ, Coleman-Minahan K. Use of judicial bypass of mandatory parental consent to access abortion and judicial bypass denials, Florida and Texas, 2018–2021. *Am J Public Health*. 2023;113(3):316–319.

Acceptance Date: November 11, 2022.

DOI: https://doi.org/10.2105/AJPH.2022.307173

CONTRIBUTORS

A. J. Stevenson conceptualized the study, complied the statistical data, and drafted the article. K. Coleman-Minahan contributed to study design, data interpretation, and the writing of the article.

ACKNOWLEDGMENTS

This work benefited from research, administrative, and computing support provided by the University of Colorado Population Center, which is funded by the Eunice Kennedy Shriver National Institute of Child Health and Human Development (project 2P2CHD066613-06). We thank Margaret Wurth of Human Rights Watch for obtaining and sharing with us official state reports on Florida's judicial bypass of parental notice and consent for abortion.

CONFLICTS OF INTEREST

The authors have no conflicts of interest to disclose.

HUMAN PARTICIPANT PROTECTION

As an analysis of aggregate public data, this study was exempt from human participant review.

REFERENCES

1. Ralph LJ, King E, Belusa E, Foster DG, Brindis CD, Biggs MA. The impact of a parental notification requirement on Illinois minors' access to and decision-making around abortion. *J Adolesc Health*. 2018;62(3):281–287. https://doi.org/10.1016/j.jadohealth.2017.09.031
2. Stevenson AJ, Coleman-Minahan K, Hays S. Denials of judicial bypass petitions for abortion in Texas before and after the 2016 bypass process change: 2001–2018. *Am J Public Health*. 2020;110(3):351–353. https://doi.org/10.2105/AJPH.2019.305491
3. Janiak E, Fulcher IR, Cottrill AA, et al. Massachusetts' parental consent law and procedural timing among adolescents undergoing abortion. *Obstet Gynecol*. 2019;133(5):978–986. https://doi.org/10.1097/AOG.0000000000003190
4. Coleman-Minahan K, Stevenson AJ, Obront E, Hays S. Adolescents obtaining abortion without parental consent: their reasons and experiences of social support. *Perspect Sex Reprod Health*. 2020;52(1):15–22. https://doi.org/10.1363/psrh.12132
5. American Academy of Pediatrics, Committee on Adolescence. The adolescent's right to confidential care when considering abortion. *Pediatrics*. 2022;150(3):e2022058780. https://doi.org/10.1542/peds.2022-058780
6. Coleman-Minahan K, Stevenson AJ, Obront E, Hays S. Young women's experiences obtaining judicial bypass for abortion in Texas. *J Adolesc Health*. 2019;64(1):20–25. https://doi.org/10.1016/j.jadohealth.2018.07.017
7. Ralph LJ, Chaiten L, Werth E, Daniel S, Brindis CD, Biggs MA. Reasons for and logistical burdens of judicial bypass for abortion in Illinois. *J Adolesc Health*. 2021;68(1):71–78. https://doi.org/10.1016/j.jadohealth.2020.08.025
8. Center for Reproductive Rights. A state-by-state alert system if Roe fell. Available at: https://reproductiverights.org/what-if-roe-fell. Accessed January 12, 2020.
9. Texas Judicial Branch. Statistics and other data: judicial bypass cases: report on disposition of judicial bypass cases by trial courts. Available at: https://www.txcourts.gov/statistics/judicial-bypass-cases. Accessed May 15, 2022.
10. Coleman-Minahan K, Stevenson AJ, Obront E, Hays S. Judicial bypass attorneys' experiences with abortion stigma in Texas courts. *Soc Sci Med*. 2021;269:113508. https://doi.org/10.1016/j.socscimed.2020.113508

School-Based Interventions to Prevent Dating and Relationship Violence and Gender-Based Violence: Systematic Review and Network Meta-Analysis

Caroline Farmer, PhD, Naomi Shaw, MSc, Andrew J. Rizzo, PhD, Noreen Orr, PhD, Annah Chollet, BA, Ann Hagell, PhD, Emma Rigby, BA, Honor Young, PhD, Vashti Berry, PhD, Chris Bonell, PhD, and G. J. Melendez-Torres, RN, DPhil, MPH

Background. Schools are sites of dating and relationship violence (DRV) and of gender-based violence (GBV) victimization and perpetration. School-based interventions can reach a broad range of students, targeting both individual and group processes that may underpin DRV and GBV. Considering DRV and GBV jointly is important because of their shared etiologies. Comparing the effectiveness of interventions using network meta-analysis (NMA) can support decision-making on optimal resource use.

Objectives. To evaluate the comparative effectiveness of school-based interventions for children aged 5 to 18 years on DRV and GBV victimization, perpetration, and related mediators.

Search Methods. We searched 21 databases in July 2020 and June 2021, alongside extensive supplementary search methods, including gray literature searches, forward and backward citation chasing, and searches on first and last author names.

Selection Criteria. We included randomized-controlled trials of interventions for children of compulsory school age implemented within the school setting, and either partially or wholly aimed at changing DRV or GBV outcomes.

Data Collection and Analysis. Pairwise meta-analyses using random-effects robust variance estimation considered intervention effectiveness on DRV and GBV victimization and perpetration using odds ratios, and on mediators (e.g., knowledge and attitudes) using standardized mean differences. Effects were divided into short-term (< 12 months postbaseline) and long-term (≥ 12 months postbaseline). NMAs on victimization and perpetration outcomes compared interventions categorized by breadth of mechanism and complexity of delivery and implementation. Meta-regression tested sensitivity to percentage of girls in the trial sample and country context.

Main Results. Our analysis included 68 trials. Evidence was stronger overall for effects on DRV than for GBV, with significant long-term impacts on DRV victimization (odds ratio [OR] = 0.82; 95% confidence interval [CI] = 0.68, 0.99) and DRV perpetration (OR = 0.78; 95% CI = 0.64, 0.94). Knowledge and attitudinal effects were predominantly short-term (e.g., for DRV-related violence acceptance, $d = 0.16$; 95% CI = 0.08, 0.24). NMAs did not suggest the superiority of any intervention type; however, most analyses for GBV outcomes were inconsistent. A higher proportion of girls in the sample was associated with increased effectiveness on long-term victimization outcomes.

Author's Conclusions. Evidence is stronger for DRV than for GBV, despite considerable heterogeneity. Certainty of findings was low or very low overall.

Public Health Implications. Violence reductions may require more than 1 school year to become apparent. More extensive interventions may not be more effective. A possible reason for stronger effectiveness for DRV is that whereas GBV is ingrained in school cultures and practices, DRV is potentially more open to change via addressing individual knowledge and attitudes. (*Am J Public Health*. 2023;113(3): 320–330. https://doi.org/10.2105/AJPH.2022.307153)

PLAIN-LANGUAGE SUMMARY

Dating and relationship violence and gender-based violence in adolescents and young people remain major issues for school health, especially given that schools are major sites for perpetration and victimization of both DRV and GBV. School-based prevention of DRV and GBV has been tested in many forms, but patterns of effectiveness across both types of outcomes have not been considered. This is especially important because of growing social awareness of how DRV and GBV are linked by toxic patriarchal norms. We searched 21 databases to find randomized trials of school-based interventions for DRV and GBV, and meta-analyzed them by short-term (< 12 months from baseline) and long-term (≥ 12 months from baseline). We included 68 trials. These trials suggested that long-term, but not short-term, impacts on victimization and perpetration for DRV were in evidence, but did not offer clear evidence of effectiveness for GBV outcomes. These trials also suggested that interventions could have short-term impacts on knowledge and attitudes, such as violence acceptance. An additional analysis that compared types of interventions did not find that more extensive (more components, broader implementation) interventions were necessarily more effective. This means that schools may need to wait longer than 1 school year to see impacts.

Conservative estimates suggest that between a quarter and a third of school-age children experience dating and relationship violence (DRV), such as physical, sexual, and psychological abuse (including online abuse and coercive control),[1] although rates of DRV in excess of two thirds of students have been reported in some contexts.[2] Students also describe gender-based violence (GBV) as "commonplace" in schools, including sexual harassment and homophobic and transphobic bullying, with sexual assaults reported in school spaces.[3] DRV and GBV share risk factors and antecedent attitudes,[4,5] including patriarchal gender norms at the societal level, inconsistently enforced violence prevention policies at the school level, and, at the individual level, exposure to and reinforcement of antisocial GBV-related norms.[1,2,6] They also share pervasive consequences for both survivors and perpetrators, including poor mental health, low self-esteem, and risky sexual behavior[2,7]; consequences for academic performance and school engagement[8,9]; and elevated risk of intimate partner violence as adults.

Schools are sites of DRV and GBV victimization and perpetration, but they are also important venues for intervention. School-based interventions can reach a broad range of students, targeting both individual and group processes that may underpin DRV and GBV.[10–12] Previous reviews[11,13,14] have evaluated the effectiveness of interventions for DRV and GBV but have not considered how these affect DRV and GBV outcomes jointly, despite overlap in antecedents. Understanding the effectiveness on both outcomes together supports greater knowledge of approaches for each outcome and informs joint implementation of interventions to reduce DRV and GBV concurrently. Several older reviews require updating to assess newer interventions, but the most recent major review[12] also missed relevant studies because of an unduly narrow approach to literature searches. Evaluations of school-based interventions are often published within gray literature (i.e., not in mainstream databases), and therefore reviews without rigorous searches of gray literature sources may exclude relevant data. Finally, to date, no previous review has undertaken a network meta-analysis (NMA) on DRV or GBV outcomes, capitalizing on a mature evidence base to estimate the comparative effectiveness of interventions. An NMA able to identify patterns in the effectiveness of interventions—such as in the breadth or level of delivery, mechanisms of action, and implementation efforts required—would be of value for policymakers seeking to select an intervention for their schools, particularly given sustained policy interest in whole-school approaches despite their complexity.[3,6] Thus, this systematic review sought to evaluate the effectiveness of school-based interventions on DRV and GBV victimization and perpetration among children aged 5 to 18 years, as well as the factors—including knowledge and attitudes—that might mediate reductions in victimization and perpetration. It also presents, for the first time, an NMA of the comparative effectiveness of intervention types on DRV and GBV victimization and perpetration.

METHODS

This review was registered on PROSPERO (CRD42020190463).

Search Methods

In July 2020, we searched the following databases without limitation on date or

AJPH March 2023, Vol 113, No. 3

language: MEDLINE, Embase, PsycINFO, Social Policy and Practice (Ovid); CINAHL, ERIC, British Education Index, Education Research Complete, EconLit, Criminal Justice Abstracts (EBSCOhost); Cochrane Database of Systematic Reviews and the Cochrane Central Register of Controlled Trials (via the Cochrane Library, Wiley); NHS Economic Evaluation Database (via the Centre for Reviews and Dissemination); Social Science Citation Index and Conference Proceedings Citation Index (Web of Science, Clarivate Analytics); Australian Education Index, ProQuest Dissertations & Theses Global, Sociological Abstracts including Social Services Abstracts, Applied Social Sciences Index and Abstracts (ProQuest); Trials Register of Promoting Health Interventions and Bibliomap (EPPI-Centre); and Campbell Systematic Reviews (Campbell Collaboration). We updated the bibliographic database searches in June 2021 and added further free-text search terms for named interventions. The timing of searches was chosen to coincide with the requirements of the funder and in preparation for submission of the funder report.

Our database searches included free-text terms and subject headings for schools and for DRV and GBV. We used forward and backward citation chasing on included studies in Scopus (Elsevier), Web of Science, and Google Scholar, and we reviewed the reference lists of relevant systematic reviews and reports. To identify linked studies and further gray literature, we conducted targeted searches in Web of Science and Scopus using first and last author names, and searched Google Scholar for specific intervention names (e.g., Project Respect, Shifting Boundaries). We also searched or browsed publication lists on key Web sites, and searched clinical trial registers (ClinicalTrials.gov, WHO ICTRP). Where missing data from trial publications was expected to affect the analysis, we contacted authors to request additional information.

All search results were downloaded into EndNote ×9 (Clarivate Analytics, London, UK) for deduplication. Further details are provided in Appendix A (available as a supplement to the online version of this article at http://www.ajph.org).

Selection Criteria

Randomized-controlled trials (RCTs) were eligible for inclusion, including cluster trials. The population was restricted to children of compulsory school age (5–18 years). Relevant interventions were implemented within the school setting (including out of school hours, provided these were conducted with school cohorts), and either partially or wholly aimed at changing DRV or GBV outcomes. We excluded interventions that might have had only opportunistic effects on DRV or GBV outcomes—for example, through another health promotion effect (e.g., healthy eating). No restriction was placed on the content of interventions, which may have involved delivery to individual or groups of students, training of staff or school personnel, and interventions targeting local and school policy changes. Interventions may have been delivered by school staff or by an external organization, or entirely peer-led (e.g., through a computerized module). Comparisons with control or other active intervention were included.

Search records were screened by 2 reviewers at both the title and abstract level and full-text level. Publications were not excluded at the title and abstract level based on outcome. Disagreements were resolved through discussion and with a third reviewer where required. A reviewer extracted data into a data extraction form developed and piloted a priori and checked by a second reviewer. Data extracted included details about the study design, study sample, intervention characteristics, analysis methods, and outcome data.

Outcomes

Outcomes included victimization or perpetration of DRV or GBV. DRV included physical violence, emotional violence (including isolation, coercive control and cyber abuse), and sexual assault within a dating relationship. Where physical and sexual DRV were considered jointly in an outcome, this was treated as a separate outcome type. GBV included violence outside of a relationship, such as harassment and bullying on the basis of gender or sexuality (including homophobic and transphobic bullying), cyber abuse (including unwanted sexting or forwarding of sexts), unwanted sexual contact (such as groping or "upskirting"), sexual assault, and rape. Trials varied in the measurement of DRV and GBV outcomes, and a pragmatic decision was taken to group together outcomes across studies based on the types of violence measured. Groupings were informed by outcome descriptions in the original studies and, where available, inspection of measurement items. For both DRV and GBV, "omnibus" measures were overall measures without differentiation (e.g., by emotional, physical, or cyber abuse). In addition, knowledge, attitudes, and behaviors related to DRV and GBV were included, such as rape myth acceptance, bystander attitudes, and GBV-condoning norms; these were grouped by similarity of construct. We did not include outcomes related to "honor"-based violence, forced marriage, or female genital cutting. Outcomes were quantitative, and included categorical, count, and continuous measures, using bespoke or validated measures. We extracted relevant moderators in included trials.

Pairwise Meta-Analysis

Analyses were based on intention-to-treat data reported by trials; per protocol data were only included if intention-to-treat analyses were not available, and were downgraded during quality appraisal. Outcomes were grouped, by length of follow-up, as short-term (< 1 year) or long-term (≥ 1 year). Pairwise meta-analyses of comparisons against control were conducted, grouped by outcome (DRV or GBV type) as per the review protocol and availability of evidence in the included trials.

The key metric for primary outcomes was the odds ratio (OR); where outcome measures were continuous, we converted these to ORs using a logistic transformation. We meta-analyzed mediators using standardized mean differences. Meta-analyses used robust variance estimation. This approach improves on previous strategies for dealing with multiple relevant effect sizes per study (e.g., from several treatment arms or effect estimates), such as artificially splitting meta-analyses or choosing 1 effect size, by including all relevant effect sizes but adjusting for interdependencies within studies.[15] As heterogeneity across study designs and interventions was anticipated, meta-analyses used a random-effects model as default. We assessed heterogeneity in part using I^2, defined as substantial (> 60%), moderate (31%–60%), little (6%–30%), and minimal (≤ 5%). For cluster trials, where the intracluster correlation coefficient was not explicitly modeled or reported, we imputed an estimate of 0.05 based on other studies used within the review, as recommended by Cochrane guidance.[16] Following adjustment, data from cluster trials were pooled with RCTs.

Network Meta-Analysis

We conducted NMAs of study effects, including trials of head-to-head comparisons, to compare the effectiveness of intervention types on DRV and GBV perpetration and victimization outcomes. On the basis of a components analysis informed by stakeholder consultation and policy priorities for school health, we grouped interventions according to delivery type, breadth of mechanism, and implementation (single-component, curriculum, multicomponent, and multilevel interventions; Table 1). We used a frequentist framework via "network" in Stata version 17 (StataCorp LP, College Station, TX). We included correlations between arms in multiarm trials using estimates from trial reports, and a common between-study variance parameter was used across the network. Because of unresolved heterogeneity in effects across trials identified in pairwise meta-analyses, only random-effects models were fitted. We explored analyses for inconsistency using design-by-treatment interaction models, and transitivity was assessed and explored by considering known effect modifiers (e.g., network meta-regression) and the similarity of interventions in each node with respect to the intervention groupings. We then ranked interventions in consistent models using 1000 bootstrap draws, with rankings summarized using the surface under the cumulative ranking curve (SUCRA). SUCRA values balance the precision of, and numerical differences between, estimates and integrate the probability of each intervention type at each rank. SUCRA values produce estimates of how interventions compare with a hypothetical situation where each intervention had 100% probability of ranking first. Where trials reported multiple effect sizes for the same outcome (e.g., different types of DRV victimization), we assumed outcomes to be correlated with $\rho = 0.8$.[15]

Quality Appraisal and Sensitivity Analysis

Two reviewers (C. F. and a research assistant) appraised all trials for quality using an adapted Cochrane risk of bias tool.[16] In the main, appraisals were guided by the tool; however, trials were not downgraded for unblinded outcome assessors within the outcome measurement domain. This decision avoided a floor effect in quality-appraisal ratings as in most trials it was infeasible for study authors to blind or obscure study aims from students. Appraisal decisions were quality assured by a third reviewer (G. J. M.-T.) and disagreements resolved through discussion. We generated comparison-adjusted funnel plots to investigate publication bias for primary outcomes. We sensitivity analyzed primary outcomes using meta-regression on country context (high-income vs low-income and middle-income) and percentage of girl children in the trial sample. These were most commonly identified by stakeholders as likely moderators of effectiveness. Pairwise meta-regressions used common between-study variance parameters between groups. Network meta-regressions additionally assumed a common coefficient across all comparisons against control.

TABLE 1— Typology of Delivery, Mechanisms, and Implementation for School-Based Interventions for Dating and Relationship Violence and Gender-Based Violence

Type	Description
Single-component interventions	
Delivery	Generally brief (e.g., 25–30 min) single sessions or a few sessions (≤5). May or may not require in-person facilitators.
Mechanisms	Focuses on a single, or very narrow range of, change mechanism.
Implementation	Often delivered through a key technology as integral to effectiveness (e.g., video game, online, immersive virtual environments).
Curriculum-based interventions	
Delivery	Generally delivered in more sessions (≥6) and over a longer term (ranging from several weeks to several years), by extensively trained external in-person facilitators following specific manuals, lesson plans, or scripts for each session.
Mechanisms	Focuses on a narrow range of change mechanisms at 1 or 2 levels but does not address higher-level (i.e., structural) change mechanisms.
Implementation	Can be integrated into existing school curriculum (personal, social, and health education, etc.) or else delivered in a classroom environment in place of existing subjects for a short period of time.
Multicomponent interventions	
Delivery	Generally delivered using a variety of modes of intervention for varying durations, including but not limited to curriculum, theater productions, videos, presentations, group and pair discussions, individual work, and the Internet.
Mechanisms	Can address multiple change mechanisms across multiple levels but does not extensively address structural change mechanisms.
Implementation	Requires some school staff investment and external facilitation.
Multilevel interventions	
Delivery	Uses a variety of modes over several ecological levels in schools, beyond just instructing students or school personnel. Integrates explicit components relating to social structural or structural environmental domains.
Mechanisms	Addresses a range of change mechanisms over multiple ecological levels.
Implementation	Requires a combination of school staff investment and external facilitation.

RESULTS

Characteristics of studies included in the review are provided in online Appendix B. Following de-duplication, we screened 40 160 records on title and abstract, and 788 records on full-text (Figure 1). Of these, we included 68 RCTs evaluating 80 interventions for DRV or GBV. These included 14 RCTs and 54 cluster RCTs that compared interventions against a control intervention (n = 66, including an active control intervention, usual practice, waitlist, or no intervention) or another active intervention (n = 8). Head-to-head comparisons were of different interventions (n = 4), of additional components (n = 3), or of different methods of implementation (n = 3). More interventions were identified as targeting DRV (n = 43) than GBV (n = 15), and 14 interventions were identified as targeting both. The intended target was unclear for 8 interventions, although these trials were included because the intervention content included topics considered relevant to either DRV or GBV.

Most studies (n = 42) were conducted in North America, with the remaining split across Europe (n = 9), Asia (n = 8), Africa (n = 6), and South America (n = 3). Across these trials, 50 were undertaken in high-income country contexts. Sample sizes ranged from 47 to 89 707 participants (median = 839). Studies were mostly conducted in middle or high schools (i.e., ages 11–18 years). Only 4 studies also or solely included students within primary or junior schools. Most trials were conducted with male and female students, whereas 4 and 6 studies, respectively, were conducted exclusively with male or female students. Only 2 studies permitted students to record gender beyond the binary, and only 5 studies included students' self-reported sexuality. No studies included solely LGBTQ+ (lesbian, gay, bisexual, transgender, or queer) students. Only half of included studies (52.9%) reported student race or ethnicity; of these, more than 50% of students identified as White or Caucasian (37.8%), Hispanic or Latino (18.9%), and Black or African American (10.8%). School or students' socioeconomic status (SES)

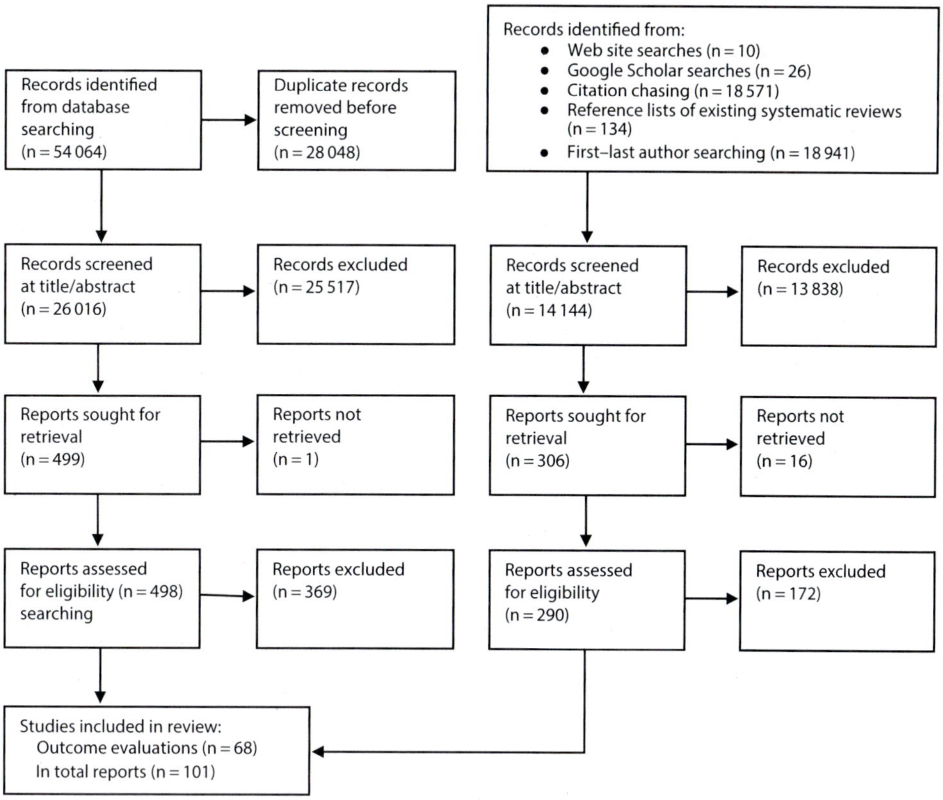

FIGURE 1— Flowchart of Studies in the Review: School-Based Interventions to Prevent Dating and Relationship Violence and Gender-Based Violence

was reported for 35 studies, of which 11 included more than 50% of students from lower SES backgrounds (e.g., free or subsidized school lunches, or in areas with high economic deprivation). No identified studies exclusively included students who had experienced DRV or GBV; however, 2 studies included only participants considered at risk for DRV.

Interventions included single-component interventions (n = 22 RCTs), curriculum interventions (n = 11), multicomponent interventions (n = 15), and multilevel interventions (n = 22). Half of all interventions included full or partial implementation by external agencies (50.1%). A minority of interventions included a self-study (12.5%) or digital (15.0%) component (e.g., use of virtual reality games). DRV and GBV interventions were not clearly different in choice of facilitator or delivery method.

Quality of Included Studies

Critical appraisals for included outcome evaluations are reported in online Appendix B. Only 1 included trial[17] was appraised at overall low risk for bias (1.5%). The other trials were split between those appraised as having "some concerns" (54.4%) and those considered to be at high risk for bias (44.1%). The main risk of bias issues in the included trials were as follows:

- unclear allocation concealment, with most trials using simple randomization procedures that can be open to manipulation;
- potential for contamination in schools where students may mix with those in other intervention arms, or teachers trained to deliver the intervention may alter their behavior toward students in the control arm; and
- loss of clusters following randomization without evidence that drop-out was unrelated to trial outcomes.

Pairwise Meta-Analyses

Pairwise meta-analyses for interventions compared with controls are reported in Table 2, with forest plots in online Appendix C. Findings suggested that school-based interventions were effective compared with controls in reducing the victimization and perpetration of DRV. A reduction in DRV was shown across subtypes of violence, and was greater at long-term follow-up. However, effect estimates were substantially

TABLE 2— Pairwise Meta-Analyses of School-Based Interventions for Dating and Relationship Violence (DRV) and Gender-Based Violence (GBV) Compared to Controls

Outcome	Short-Term Follow-Up (< 1 y)				Long-Term Follow-Up (≥ 1 y)			
	k	No.	OR (95% CI)	I^2 (%)	k	No.	OR (95% CI)	I^2 (%)
DRV victimization								
All outcomes	17	118	0.90 (0.80, 1.02)	81	13	79	0.82 (0.68, 0.99)	80
Omnibus	10	45	0.88 (0.69, 1.12)	84	5	12	0.85 (0.63, 1.15)	52
Emotional/psychological	8	16	0.84 (0.55, 1.27)	90	9	21	0.81 (0.59, 1.12)	88
Physical	5	14	0.93 (0.69, 1.25)	64	6	21	0.84 (0.61, 1.16)	82
Sexual	7	29	0.97 (0.88, 1.08)	76	5	13	0.88 (0.59, 1.31)	78
Physical/sexual	4	8	0.85 (0.43, 1.69)	76	5	9	0.90 (0.53, 1.51)	73
Cyber	3	6	0.82 (0.31, 2.16)	87	2	3	0.57 (0.45, 0.72)	0
DRV perpetration								
All outcomes	18	118	0.91 (0.80, 1.04)	83	16	79	0.78 (0.64, 0.94)	79
Omnibus	11	43	0.95 (0.85, 1.07)	70	7	15	0.74 (0.52, 1.06)	75
Emotional/psychological	9	19	0.77 (0.54, 1.11)	90	9	21	0.77 (0.59, 1.01)	85
Physical	7	16	0.91 (0.71, 1.18)	83	7	22	0.83 (0.59, 1.18)	80
Sexual	7	30	0.99 (0.86, 1.13)	79	4	9	0.85 (0.37, 1.92)	60
Physical/sexual	3	6	0.82 (0.13, 5.29)	76	5	9	0.77 (0.42, 1.43)	78
Cyber	2	4	0.96 (0.77, 1.18)	71	2	3	0.49 (0.38, 0.63)	50
GBV victimization								
All outcomes	13	72	0.88 (0.76, 1.02)	75	11	58	0.93 (0.80, 1.08)	66
Omnibus	7	29	1.00 (0.91, 1.10)	60	7	17	0.93 (0.79, 1.10)	41
Emotional/verbal	2	2	0.94 (0.82, 1.08)	0	3	11	0.92 (0.56, 1.52)	76
Physical	9	40	0.76 (0.62, 0.93)	78	6	25	0.91 (0.68, 1.23)	66
Homophobic	1	1	1.01 (0.77, 1.33)	...	1	5	(Not estimable)	
GBV perpetration								
All outcomes	11	67	0.95 (0.85, 1.07)	66	9	58	0.90 (0.73, 1.12)	67
Omnibus	9	30	0.97 (0.88, 1.06)	55	6	15	0.98 (0.73, 1.30)	57
Emotional/verbal	2	2	0.85 (0.40, 1.80)	76	4	12	0.86 (0.60, 1.24)	63
Physical	5	33	0.87 (0.62, 1.23)	77	5	24	0.79 (0.48, 1.28)	68
Homophobic	2	2	1.06 (0.85, 1.32)	0	2	7	0.95 (0.89, 1.02)	38

Note. CI = confidence interval; OR = odds ratio.

heterogeneous, with wide confidence intervals (CIs) typically crossing the line of null effect. School-based interventions may be effective for reducing victimization and perpetration of GBV; however, effects were smaller than for DRV, and all effects were highly imprecise. Findings were similar across subtypes of GBV, and heterogeneity was also substantial in these analyses. GRADE for pairwise meta-analyses (Appendix C) led to all outcomes rated as low or very low certainty of evidence, owing primarily to substantial unexplained heterogeneity and risk of publication bias.

Meta-regression sensitivity analyses (Appendix C) also showed that country context moderated effects for DRV or GBV, particularly at long-term follow-up. At 1 year or longer after baseline, interventions in high-income contexts were associated with larger reductions in the odds of DRV and GBV victimization and perpetration (ORs = 0.71–0.86; all *Ps* < .05). Furthermore, the proportion of girls in the trial sample moderated effects for DRV and GBV victimization, but not for DRV or GBV perpetration. With each additional 10% points of girls in the sample, the odds of DRV victimization decreased by 22% (although the effect was marginally nonsignificant; OR = 0.78; 95% CI = 0.59, 1.04) and the odds of GBV victimization decreased by 9% (OR = 0.91; 95% CI = 0.85, 0.97).

Analyses of Knowledge and Attitudes

Meta-analyses of knowledge and attitudes are presented in online Appendix C. Overall, interventions were effective at improving short-term DRV-focused violence acceptance (d = 0.16; 95% CI = 0.08, 0.24), knowledge (d = 0.69; 95% CI = 0.18, 1.20), attitudes to intervening (d = 0.14; 95% CI = 0.01, 0.26), and attitudes to personal help-seeking (d = 0.14; 95% CI = 0.06, 0.22), but none of these effects was maintained in long-term analyses. Interventions improved GBV-focused violence acceptance (d = 0.29; 95% CI = 0.11, 0.33), knowledge (d = 0.68; 95% CI = 0.26, 1.11), and individual self-efficacy (d = 0.16; 95% CI = 0.08, 0.25) in the short term, with only violence acceptance having a credible long-term effect.

Network Meta-Analyses

NMA findings (Table 3) suggested that single-component interventions may be useful for reducing short-term and long-term DRV victimization and perpetration, and also short-term GBV victimization (no single-component interventions were tested in long-term GBV victimization). Multilevel interventions also showed effectiveness for long-term DRV victimization. For GBV outcomes, there was strongest evidence for curriculum interventions, which were more successful than other intervention types at short-term follow-up of victimization and short-term and long-term perpetration. Consistency tests for short-term DRV outcomes yielded no evidence of inconsistency (victimization: $\chi^2 = 0.29$, $df = 3$, $P = .96$; perpetration: $\chi^2 = 0.16$, $df = 3$, $P = .98$). However, inconsistency tests were significant for all GBV analyses except for short-term GBV victimization ($\chi^2 = 7.24$, $df = 3$, $P = .06$), driven primarily by 1 trial.

Assessment of transitivity suggested that interventions were more similar within node than between node, but effect modifiers (specifically, country context and sex) were explored to evaluate the impact of imbalances (Appendix C). These analyses had minimal effect on DRV outcomes. However, accounting for the percentage of girls in the trial sample led to comparable effectiveness for short-term GBV victimization across intervention types (although no effect at long-term). Controlling for country context did not affect short-term GBV victimization or perpetration, although in long-term analyses curriculum interventions became more effective.

Rank data are presented in full in Appendix C for consistent NMAs. Overall, single-component interventions were most likely to be top-ranked for DRV victimization and perpetration (SUCRA = 0.8–1.0). Curriculum interventions were most likely to be top-ranked for GBV victimization in the short term (SUCRA = 0.9).

Publication Bias Analyses

Funnel plots (Appendix C) showed evidence of publication bias in short-term DRV victimization, DRV perpetration, and GBV victimization, and in long-term DRV perpetration and GBV victimization. In most cases, bias was toward publication of positive intervention effects by smaller trials, although for GBV victimization, smaller trials were more likely to report negative effects.

DISCUSSION

The results of this comprehensive systematic review and meta-analysis of school-based interventions for DRV and GBV suggest that evidence for the effectiveness of school-based interventions is stronger for DRV than for GBV. However, effects may not be immediate and may require more than 1 school year to become apparent. Effects are evident in the aggregate rather than for any specific type of DRV or GBV. This is an advantage of our analysis strategy, which used an innovative statistical method to integrate all relevant evidence. Interventions are also linked with primarily short-term effects on knowledge and attitudinal mediators. Our consideration of mediators is the most exhaustive to date. It is possible that, whereas effects on mediators may have faded after short-term measurement, longer-term behavior change occurred via changes in school social systems, practices, and norms that may be less amenable to measurement in terms of knowledge and attitudes.

However, there are some caveats in this body of evidence. First, there were clear differences in the sufficiency of evidence for different types of violence. For example, homophobic GBV was evaluated in very few trials, despite clear evidence of DRV and GBV inequalities in sexual-minority groups.[18] Moreover, most GBV analyses relied on omnibus measures that did not distinguish between types of violence. Very few studies reported data for groups at higher risk for DRV or GBV—for example, those with experience of violence, or sexual minorities.[19] In addition, publication bias was assessed as a serious risk for several of the victimization and perpetration outcomes.

NMAs for most GBV outcomes were inconsistent, limiting interpretation of this evidence. Specifically, inconsistency in NMAs derived from conflicts between trials comparing different intervention

TABLE 3— Network Meta-Analyses of School-Based Interventions for Dating and Relationship Violence (DRV) and Gender-Based Violence (GBV), by Intervention Typology

	Short-Term Follow-Up, OR (95% CI)				Long-Term Follow-Up, OR (95% CI)			
	Single	Curriculum	Multicomponent	Multilevel	Single	Curriculum	Multicomponent	Multilevel
DRV victimization								
Control	0.88 (0.75, 1.03)	0.97 (0.70, 1.34)	1.01 (0.84, 1.22)	0.89 (0.76, 1.05)	0.60 (0.41, 0.86)	0.92 (0.61, 1.40)	0.94 (0.73, 1.20)	0.83 (0.69, 1.00)
Single		1.10 (0.77, 1.57)	1.15 (0.90, 1.47)	1.02 (0.81, 1.27)		1.54 (0.88, 2.69)	1.57 (1.01, 2.45)	1.39 (0.92, 2.10)
Curriculum			1.04 (0.72, 1.51)	0.92 (0.69, 1.24)			1.02 (0.63, 1.66)	0.90 (0.62, 1.31)
Multicomponent				0.88 (0.70, 1.11)				0.88 (0.65, 1.21)
DRV perpetration								
Control	0.81 (0.65, 1.02)	0.90 (0.68, 1.19)	0.99 (0.79, 1.24)	0.87 (0.70, 1.08)	0.57 (0.40, 0.83)	0.97 (0.63, 1.50)	0.83 (0.65, 1.06)	0.86 (0.69, 1.06)
Single		1.11 (0.78, 1.58)	1.22 (0.89, 1.68)	1.07 (0.79, 1.45)		1.69 (0.94, 3.02)	1.44 (0.90, 2.29)	1.49 (0.96, 2.32)
Curriculum			1.10 (0.78, 1.56)	0.96 (0.72, 1.29)			0.85 (0.53, 1.37)	0.88 (0.61, 1.29)
Multicomponent				0.87 (0.66, 1.17)				1.04 (0.77, 1.39)
GBV victimization								
Control	0.87 (0.66, 1.14)	0.72 (0.54, 0.95)	0.95 (0.77, 1.16)	0.90 (0.75, 1.09)	. . .	0.93 (0.66, 1.32)	0.89 (0.75, 1.07)	0.95 (0.77, 1.18)
Single		0.83 (0.57, 1.21)	1.09 (0.78, 1.53)	1.04 (0.74, 1.46)		. . .	. . .	. . .
Curriculum			1.32 (0.94, 1.85)	1.26 (0.94, 1.69)			0.96 (0.67, 1.37)	1.02 (0.69, 1.53)
Multicomponent				0.95 (0.74, 1.23)				1.07 (0.80, 1.44)
GBV perpetration								
Control	1.00 (0.90, 1.11)	0.88 (0.70, 1.10)	0.95 (0.85, 1.06)	0.89 (0.78, 1.02)	. . .	0.82 (0.54, 1.26)	0.89 (0.70, 1.14)	0.95 (0.72, 1.25)
Single		0.88 (0.69, 1.11)	0.95 (0.81, 1.11)	0.89 (0.75, 1.07)		. . .	. . .	. . .
Curriculum			1.08 (0.83, 1.41)	1.02 (0.83, 1.25)			1.08 (0.66, 1.76)	1.15 (0.79, 1.68)
Multicomponent				0.94 (0.81, 1.09)				1.07 (0.74, 1.54)

Note. CI = confidence interval; OR = odds ratio. Ellipses denote "not applicable."

types directly and trials comparing each intervention type against control. This again suggests that evidence supporting the effectiveness of interventions was stronger for DRV than for GBV. GBV victimization and perpetration effectiveness was also moderated by country context. Although this did suggest that interventions were effective for GBV in high-income contexts, these analyses relied on relatively few studies and meta-regressions are not causal. Future evaluations should also consider our findings related to the proportion of girls in trial samples and its relationship to victimization outcomes. Interventions addressed to mixed-sex audiences could only show effectiveness because of the positive effects on girls' victimization, rather than on adolescents' perpetration. This is important because decreases in victimization do not suggest specifically that primary prevention of violence is occurring, only that the violence being committed by anyone in the sample is (postintervention) more often directed outside of the sample.

Strengths and Limitations

Compared with prior reviews, our analysis has several strengths. First, the extensive and wide-ranging search permitted a clearer perspective as to the effectiveness of interventions on a range of mediators. Moreover, we were able to include a number of RCTs, including in the gray literature, that previous reviews have not included. Second, our joint consideration of DRV and GBV highlights an important gap in the evidence that requires further consideration; specifically, why intervention impacts appear stronger for DRV than for GBV.

However, our analysis has several limitations. First, we cannot exclude the possibility that relevant trials were missed either because of database indexing or the "file drawer problem," and indeed, our analysis of publication bias indicates some risk of this. Second, we did not analyze broader gender norms and related constructs (e.g., homophobia generally), given the need to identify clear inclusion and exclusion criteria. Third, substantial heterogeneity in intervention effects reflected that variation between interventions could not be explained by our intervention typology, or by variation in potential effect modifiers such as sample demographics, outcome measurement, or trial design. This suggests the need for careful consideration of fit between interventions and local contexts before implementing, and the possibility that explanations for heterogeneity arise from configurations of conditions and components rather than individual predictors. Finally, we adapted the Cochrane risk of bias tool to avoid a floor effect in quality-appraisal ratings across trials. This decision allowed greater comparison of quality across included studies, but the lack of blinding is nevertheless a significant risk of bias in the evidence base.

Implications for Policy and Practice

This is the first published systematic review in this area to compare different intervention types via NMA. Our classification strategy, led by stakeholder consultation suggesting the importance of understanding intervention breadth and difficulty of implementation, led to a surprising finding: that more extensive interventions targeting a broader range of system levels, stakeholders, and change mechanisms were not necessarily more effective than single-component (and frequently technologically mediated) interventions. A possible reason for this relates to school capacity to implement complex interventions,[20] such that the effectiveness of single-component interventions may be related to the relative ease of rigorous implementation. This finding may be significant for schools seeking to deliver an intervention for DRV or GBV to students, but with limited resources for complex, multilevel interventions.

Our analysis raises important questions about why interventions might be more effective—and more consistently effective—for DRV. A possible reason for this is that, whereas GBV is immanent and ingrained in school cultures and practices, DRV is a more private behavior[3] and potentially more open to change via addressing individual knowledge and attitudes. Similarly, given rapid turnover in adolescent dating relationships, young people may have more opportunities to alter relationship dynamics in ways not present for GBV, given that peer relationships may be less amenable to change.

Future trials and reviews should incorporate outcomes beyond individual behaviors, knowledge, or attitudes. Although these are useful at gauging intervention impacts on individuals, they do not capture the broader system and community effects of an intervention,[21] which were not evidenced in our review. In addition, our findings suggest that interventions may require several years of implementation to show meaningful impacts for DRV and GBV. This may be a barrier for many schools given short-term improvement targets. Schools should consider preintervention implementation work to integrate delivery and maintenance of an intervention into existing school practices, and to maximize the public health benefits of implemented interventions. AJPH

ABOUT THE AUTHORS

Caroline Farmer, Naomi Shaw, Noreen Orr, Vashti Berry, and G. J. Melendez-Torres are with the Faculty of Health and Life Sciences, University of Exeter, Exeter, UK. Andrew J. Rizzo is with the College of Health and Human Performance, University of Florida, Gainesville. Annah Chollet is with the Department of Social Policy and Intervention, University of Oxford, Oxford, UK. Ann Hagell and Emma Rigby are with the Association for Young People's Health, London, UK. Honor Young is with the Centre for Development, Evaluation, Complexity and Implementation in Public Health Improvement (DECIPHer), Cardiff University, Cardiff, UK. Chris Bonell is with the Department of Public Health Environments and Society, London School of Hygiene and Tropical Medicine, London, UK.

CORRESPONDENCE

Correspondence should be sent to G. J. Melendez-Torres, Faculty of Health and Life Sciences, University of Exeter, EX1 2LU, Exeter, UK (e-mail: g.j.melendez-torres@exeter.ac.uk). Reprints can be ordered at http://www.ajph.org by clicking the "Reprints" link.

PUBLICATION INFORMATION

Full Citation: Farmer C, Shaw N, Rizzo AJ, et al. School-based interventions to prevent dating and relationship violence and gender-based violence: systematic review and network meta-analysis. *Am J Public Health*. 2023;113(3):320–330.

Acceptance Date: October 13, 2022.

DOI: https://doi.org/10.2105/AJPH.2022.307153

CONTRIBUTORS

C. Farmer, N. Shaw, and G. J. Melendez-Torres conceptualized and designed the study, collected the data, drafted the initial manuscript, and reviewed and revised the manuscript. A. J. Rizzo, N. Orr, and A. Chollet collected the data, contributed to interpretation, and reviewed and revised the manuscript. A. Hagell, E. Rigby, H. Young, V. Berry, and C. Bonell contributed to interpretation and reviewed and revised the manuscript.

ACKNOWLEDGMENTS

This study is funded by the National Institute for Health Research (NIHR) Public Health Research Programme (NIHR130144). In addition, V. Berry and G. J. Melendez-Torres are partly supported by the NIHR Applied Research Collaboration South West Peninsula (NIHR PenARC) and Chris Bonell is partly funded by an NIHR senior investigator award.

We gratefully acknowledge the assistance of Fraizer Kiff with study appraisal.

Note. The views expressed are those of the authors and not necessarily those of the NIHR or the Department of Health and Social Care. The funders had no role in the design and conduct of the study.

CONFLICTS OF INTEREST

C. Bonell was the principal investigator, and H. Young and G. J. Melendez-Torres co-investigators, of one of the trials included in this meta-analysis.

HUMAN PARTICIPANT PROTECTION

This research did not require ethics approval as it was based on publicly available data. However, ethics approval from the University of Exeter (ID 488499) was received to access and generate summary descriptive statistics from 2 data sets (ICPSR 22660, ICPSR 36355).

REFERENCES

1. Young H, Long SJ, Melendez-Torres GJ, et al. Dating and relationship violence victimization and perpetration among 11–16 year olds in Wales: a cross-sectional analysis of the School Health Research Network (SHRN) survey. *J Public Health (Oxf)*. 2021;43(1):111–122. https://doi.org/10.1093/pubmed/fdz084
2. Taquette SR, Monteiro DLM. Causes and consequences of adolescent dating violence: a systematic review. *J Inj Violence Res*. 2019;11(2):137–147. https://doi.org/10.5249/jivr.v11i2.1061
3. Office for Standards in Education, Children's Services and Skills (Ofsted). Review of sexual abuse in schools and colleges. 2021. Available at: https://www.gov.uk/government/publications/review-of-sexual-abuse-in-schools-and-colleges/review-of-sexual-abuse-in-schools-and-colleges. Accessed May 17, 2022.
4. Exner-Cortens D, Eckenrode J, Bunge J, Rothman E. Revictimization after adolescent dating violence in a matched, national sample of youth. *J Adolesc Health*. 2017;60(2):176–183. https://doi.org/10.1016/j.jadohealth.2016.09.015
5. Exner-Cortens D, Eckenrode J, Rothman E. Longitudinal associations between teen dating violence victimization and adverse health outcomes. *Pediatrics*. 2013;131(1):71–78. https://doi.org/10.1542/peds.2012-1029
6. Earnest AA, Brady SS. Dating violence victimization among high school students in Minnesota: associations with family violence, unsafe schools, and resources for support. *J Interpers Violence*. 2014;31(3):383–406. https://doi.org/10.1177/0886260514555863
7. Bendixen M, Daveronis J, Kennair LEO. The effects of non-physical peer sexual harassment on high school students' psychological well-being in Norway: consistent and stable findings across studies. *Int J Public Health*. 2018;63(1):3–11. https://doi.org/10.1007/s00038-017-1049-3
8. Chronister KM, Marsiglio MC, Linville D, Lantrip KR. The influence of dating violence on adolescent girls' educational experiences. *Couns Psychol*. 2013;42(3):374–405. https://doi.org/10.1177/0011000012470569
9. Aragon SR, Poteat VP, Espelage DL, Koenig BW. The influence of peer victimization on educational outcomes for LGBTQ and non-LGBTQ high school students. *J LGBT Youth*. 2014;11(1):1–19. https://doi.org/10.1080/19361653.2014.840761
10. Fellmeth GLT, Heffernan C, Nurse J, Habibula S, Sethi D. Educational and skills-based interventions for preventing relationship and dating violence in adolescents and young adults. *Cochrane Database Syst Rev*. 2013;(6):CD004534. https://doi.org/10.1002/14651858.CD004534.pub3
11. Kettrey HH, Marx RA, Tanner-Smith EE. Effects of bystander programs on the prevention of sexual assault among adolescents and college students: a systematic review. *Campbell Syst Rev*. 2019;15(1–2):e1013. https://doi.org/10.4073/csr.2019.1
12. Piolanti A, Foran HM. Efficacy of interventions to prevent physical and sexual dating violence among adolescents: a systematic review and meta-analysis. *JAMA Pediatr*. 2022;176(2):142–149. https://doi.org/10.1001/jamapediatrics.2021.4829
13. De La Rue L, Polanin JR, Espelage DL, Pigott TD. A meta-analysis of school-based interventions aimed to prevent or reduce violence in teen dating relationships. *Rev Educ Res*. 2016;87(1):7–34. https://doi.org/10.3102/0034654316632061
14. Stanley N, Ellis J, Farrelly N, Hollinghurst S, Downe S. Preventing domestic abuse for children and young people: a review of school-based interventions. *Child Youth Serv Rev*. 2015;59:120–131. https://doi.org/10.1016/j.childyouth.2015.10.018
15. Tanner-Smith EE, Tipton E. Robust variance estimation with dependent effect sizes: practical considerations including a software tutorial in Stata and SPSS. https://doi.org/10.1002/jrsm.1091. *Res Synth Methods*. 2014;5(1):13–30.
16. Higgins JPT, Thomas J, Chandler J, et al., eds. *Cochrane Handbook for Systematic Reviews of Interventions*. 2nd ed. Oxford, UK: John Wiley & Sons; 2019. https://doi.org/10.1002/9781119536604
17. Meiksin R, Crichton J, Dodd M, et al. A school intervention for 13- to 15-year-olds to prevent dating and relationship violence: the Project Respect pilot cluster RCT. *Public Health Res*. 2020;8(5):1–338. https://doi.org/10.3310/phr08050
18. Olsen EOM, Vivolo-Kantor A, Kann L. Physical and sexual teen dating violence victimization and sexual identity among US high school students, 2015. *J Interpers Violence*. 2020;35(17–18):3581–3600. https://doi.org/10.1177/0886260517708757
19. Blondeel K, de Vasconcelos S, Garcia-Moreno C, Stephenson R, Temmerman M, Toskin I. Violence motivated by perception of sexual orientation and gender identity: a systematic review. *Bull World Health Organ*. 2018;96(1):29L–41L. https://doi.org/10.2471/BLT.17.197251
20. Moore GF, Evans RE, Hawkins J, et al. From complex social interventions to interventions in complex social systems: future directions and unresolved questions for intervention development and evaluation. *Evaluation*. 2019/01/01 2019;25(1):23–45. https://doi.org/10.1177/1356389018803219
21. Burnham J, Banyard V, Ast RS, Edwards KM. Case study of community-level domestic and sexual violence prevention: using concept mapping to evaluate community narratives over time. *J Fam Violence*. 2022;37(1):43–57. https://doi.org/10.1007/s10896-021-00296-z

Dollar Stores and Food Access for Rural Households in the United States, 2008–2020

Wenhui Feng, PhD, MPP, Elina T. Page, PhD, MS, and Sean B. Cash, PhD, MA, MS

Dollar stores have rapidly expanded their food offerings in recent years. These foods tend to be higher in calories and lower in nutrients, raising public health concerns, especially in rural and low-income areas where food-access challenges are often greatest. However, there is limited empirical evidence evaluating the impact of this expansion on household food purchases on a national scale.

Using data from a yearly, nationally representative panel of approximately 50 000 households, we estimated the share of food purchases from 2008 to 2020 by store type and evaluated the role of dollar stores as food retailers in the United States.

We found that dollar stores were the fastest-growing food retailers by household expenditure share (increasing by 89.7%), with rural growth outpacing growth elsewhere (increasing by 102.9%). Though dollar stores still represent a small share of national household food purchases (2.1% in 2020), they play an increasingly prominent role in food-at-home purchases for certain disadvantaged and rural communities. Understanding the quality of the foods they offer and how this may affect diet-related health outcomes is warranted. (*Am J Public Health*. 2023;113(3):331–336. https://doi.org/10.2105/AJPH.2022.307193)

AJPH March 2023, Vol 113, No. 3

The absolute number of grocery stores in the United States has been declining since the Great Recession. Supercenters and dollar stores have picked up most of the lost shares of grocery stores, especially in rural areas.[1] In particular, dollar stores, traditionally viewed as a destination for discount purchases, offer foods that are mostly packaged, shelf-stable, higher in calories, and lower in nutrients.[2] In recent years, dollar stores have rapidly expanded their retail footprint in ways that are highly visible in communities across the country,[3] yet there is limited empirical evidence investigating the impact of this expansion on household food purchases on a national scale.

Rural communities especially face a substantial challenge with regard to food access. Rural areas have significantly fewer food retailers than urban areas,[4] and rural households with lower incomes are likely to be located farther from the closest food stores.[5] Some studies have found that increased access to healthy foods is associated with better health outcomes at the community level, including lower levels of obesity.[6,7] However, findings on this relationship are mixed, and the evidence on causal pathways is inconclusive.[8,9] Given that rural populations have higher baseline levels of obesity,[10] food access and the healthfulness of food purchases in rural areas are of great public health interest. In this study, we analyzed the role of dollar stores as food retailers in rural areas of the United States and the impact on food purchases for at-home consumption. Our results showed that there is substantial growth of dollar stores in the food retail landscape.

METHODS

The primary data set used in this analysis was the Information Resources Inc (IRI) Consumer Network, a yearly, nationally representative panel of approximately 50 000 households that provide a detailed account of their retail food purchases, including both perishable, random-weight items and consumer packaged goods. We included all currently available years of data (2008–2020) in this analysis. The Consumer Network differentiates purchases made at different store types (e.g., grocery stores, drug stores, and mass merchandisers) and includes dollar stores as a retail channel category. We applied survey sample weights (projection15K) to be geographically and demographically representative of the contiguous United States.

To assess the rurality of households participating in the panel, we matched and merged household zip-code data with rural–urban commuting area (RUCA) codes developed by the US Department of Agriculture.[11] These codes, based on data from the 2010 Decennial Census and the 2006–2010 American Community Survey, classify US census tracts using measures of population density, urbanization, and daily commuting. We categorized communities into 4 groups based on the primary RUCA codes: metropolitan (1–3), micropolitan (4–6), small town (7–9), and rural (10).

Finally, we aggregated household food expenditures by household, store type, and year. We classified store types the same way as IRI: grocery stores, drug stores, mass merchandisers, supercenters, convenience stores, dollar stores, club stores, and other. For the purposes of this analysis, we excluded nonfood items, such as liquor and tobacco products. We also dropped purchases of food items with single-trip costs beyond $500, as these were more likely to be reporting errors or purchases not intended for regular household consumption (e.g., purchasing snacks for an event) or other nontypical shopping events. The use of a $500 cutoff in this study is ultimately an arbitrary one, but we note that it only removed 0.02% (i.e., 1/50 of 1%) of shopping trips for 2008 to 2020.

Our main variable of interest was the share of food expenditures in dollar stores. We first show how food expenditure shares changed from 2008 to 2020, compared with other store types, for all regions and for rural regions; we assessed statistical significance of these changes through an analysis of variance test for each store type treating time as a categorical variable. We then further analyzed dollar store expenditure shares by rurality as well as by income, race and ethnicity, and region.

RESULTS

Figure 1 shows the change in household food expenditure shares by each

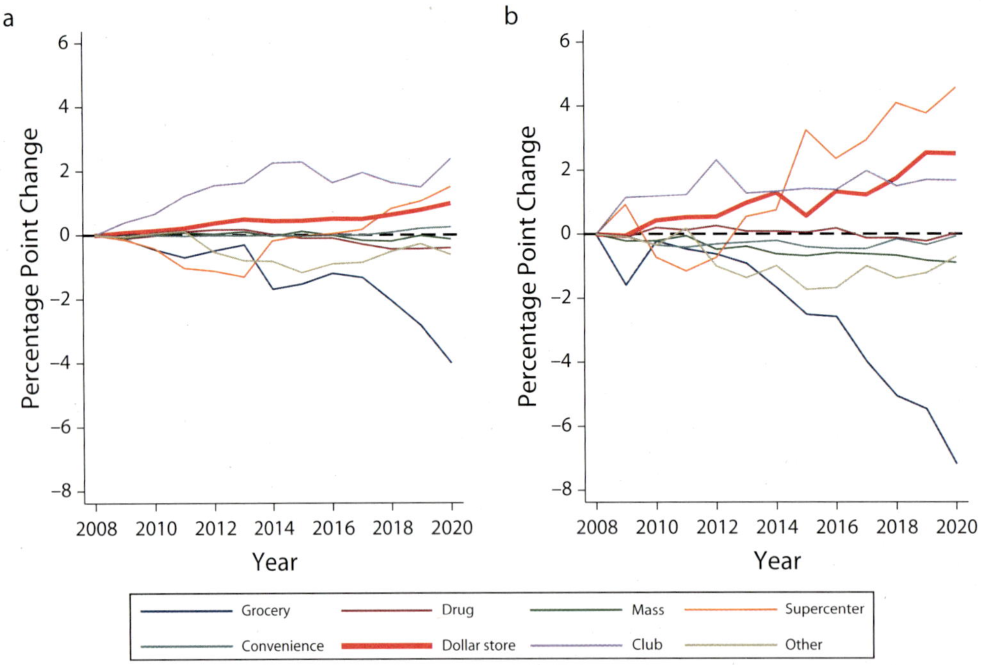

FIGURE 1— Change of Share of Household Food Spending in Dollar Stores and Other Formats for (a) All Regions Including Rural and (b) Rural Regions Only: United States, 2008–2020

Note. Projection factors (projection15k) applied to be representative of the US population. "Rural" includes households coded as such by US Department of Agriculture rural–urban commuting area classifications (i.e., primary code 10).
Source. Authors' analysis of the Information Resources Inc (IRI) Consumer Network data. The values graphed are available in Appendix A (available as a supplement to the online version of this article at https://ajph.org).

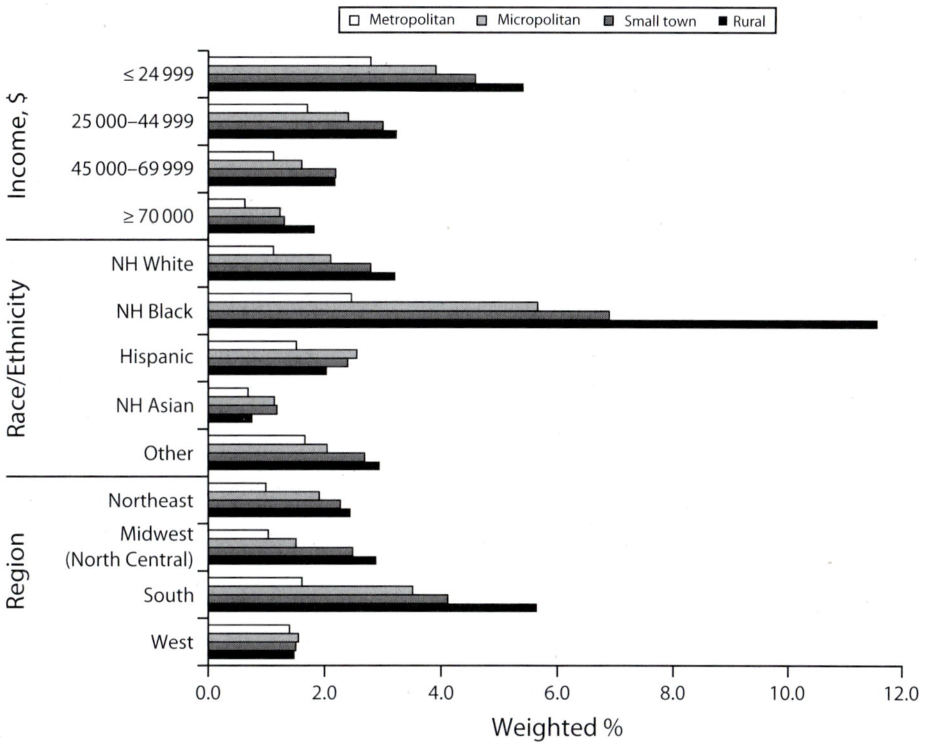

FIGURE 2— Share of Household Food Spending in Dollar Stores by Income, Race and Ethnicity, and Region: United States, 2008–2020

Note. NH = non-Hispanic. Projection factors (projection15k) applied to be representative of the US population. We categorized communities into 4 groups based on US Department of Agriculture rural–urban commuting area classifications: metropolitan (1–3), micropolitan (4–6), small town (7–9), and rural (10).
Source. Authors' analysis of the Information Resources Inc (IRI) Consumer Network data. The values graphed are available in Appendix B (available as a supplement to the online version of this article at https://ajph.org).

store type, for all regions as well as just rural regions, from 2008 to 2020; complete statistics on the absolute food expenditure shares by store type and year are provided in Appendix A (available as a supplement to the online version of this article at https://ajph.org). All changes were highly statistically significant ($P < .001$). In 2008, households spent an average of 62.3% of their food budget in grocery stores. This number declined to 58.3% in 2020. This loss was picked up by club stores (2.4 percentage points), supercenters (1.5 percentage points), dollar stores (1.0 percentage point), and convenience stores (0.2 percentage point). Dollar stores were the fastest-growing retail channel (increasing their share of household food purchases by 89.7%), followed by convenience stores (47.6%) and club stores (30.8%).

Among households living in rural areas, expenditure shares at grocery stores decreased from 57.4% in 2008 to 50.3% in 2020. This loss was picked up mostly by supercenters (4.6 percentage points), dollar stores (2.5 percentage points), and club stores (1.7 percentage points). Notably, household spending at dollar stores in rural areas increased from 2.5% in 2008 to 5.0% in 2020. In fact, dollar stores were the fastest-growing food-retail channel in rural areas (increasing their share of household food purchases by 102.9%), followed by club stores (49.2%) and supercenters (18.5%). Although supercenters gained a greater share in terms of absolute value, dollar stores increased the most by relative magnitude, doubling their share in household expenditures.

Figure 2 shows the distribution of food expenditure in dollars by urbanicity and a few key demographic indicators. Rural households purchased more foods in dollar stores across almost all demographic groups. The exceptions were rural Hispanic and non-Hispanic Asian households, for whom the sample size might be too small from which to draw meaningful conclusions (Appendix B, available as a supplement to the online version of this article at https://ajph.org). As income decreased, the share of food expenditures in dollar stores increased. Households in the South also purchased more food in dollar stores; within rural areas, households in the South spent the most, and those in the West spent the least. Perhaps the most notable group was rural non-Hispanic Black shoppers; these households spent 11.6% of their food budgets in dollar stores.

DISCUSSION

Food purchases in rural areas over the past decade are largely characterized by a shift in expenditures away from grocery stores toward both larger supercenters and smaller dollar stores. Our focus here is on the latter because of the concerns posed by how the foods dollar stores carry differ from those in traditional grocery stores; more research is needed to ascertain whether and how this evolution has also changed the nature of the foods being purchased by consumers.

Dollar stores have experienced the greatest growth in household food purchases over the past decade in terms of relative magnitude, having doubled their market share in rural areas. This rapid growth of dollar stores across the United States since the Great Recession has largely been driven by the rapid expansion of 3 major national chains, which have primarily opened stores in small, rural towns with limited retail options. One chain, Dollar General, planned to open 1100 stores in 2022.[12]

The concerns surrounding dollar stores and food access center around selection and healthfulness.[13] The selection of foods available in dollar stores is typically both less diverse and less healthful than what is found in grocery stores. Historically, dollar stores have only carried shelf-stable beverages and snacks, but now many also carry eggs and dairy, and, more recently, select locations also carry fresh produce.[14] Such changes may also partially explain the observed increase in household food purchases at these outlets. Public health advocates have raised concerns that the foods sold in dollar stores are mostly packaged, higher in calories, and lower in nutrients.[15,16] Several studies support these claims; they have found that the foods and beverages sold in dollar stores tend to be lower in nutrients and higher in calories.[2,4]

The recent growth in dollar store food expenditures along with the decline in grocery store food spending, particularly in rural areas, raises concerns that dollar stores may challenge and force out local grocers through competitive pricing, leaving consumers with limited, less-healthy food options. Several localities have already acted on the basis of these concerns. Twenty-five local governments across the country have established policies to curb the expansion of dollar stores. Among them, 9 have specified exemptions if a new dollar store provides certain levels of access to fresh food and produce.[17]

Alternatively, dollar stores may be filling food voids where local grocers do not have enough business to support maintaining a store,[18] providing consumers with food options in low-access areas. Similarly, grocery stores' consolidation may also leave residents with fewer food options, especially in rural areas.[19] In communities where other food storefronts are much farther away, dollar stores may be the only option in terms of food access.

Future Work

Although both characterizations of the impact of dollar stores on food acquisition may be sensible theoretically, empirical evidence is still lacking. Further research is needed to explore the full impact of dollar stores in areas with low food access and their impact on health and health equity. Our findings suggest that dollar stores are a significant food source for certain disadvantaged populations, especially non-Hispanic Black households in rural areas. We hope our study can instigate more conversation about the role of dollar stores in the food retail landscape and food access across subpopulations.

The lack of studies may partially be explained by the lack of data on food purchases over an extended period. Traditional survey methods, such as the National Health and Nutrition Examination Survey, rely on recall of food purchase and consumption, which may be prone to bias and only captures brief windows of time.[20] Innovative methods or the usage of underutilized data sets can create a pathway for future studies in this direction.

Limitations

This study does have a few limitations. Despite the richness of the IRI Consumer Network data, its sampling strategy is focused on metropolitan areas, leaving the sample size relatively small in rural areas. Similarly, the panel of participants in the IRI data overrepresents non-Hispanic White persons. Interpretation of results pertaining to certain racial minorities (e.g., non-Hispanic Asian persons), especially those in rural areas, should be done with caution. The available data capture a broad variety of shopping trips, and it is not obvious a priori how to distinguish household food shopping trips from those purchases of food by Consumer Network participants that may not be for "typical" household consumption. At the same time, the data also only capture purchases from stores, while nonretail acquisitions such as informal exchanges and community-based meals cannot be assessed, which may be an important part of food consumption for many rural households.[21]

Our analysis also does not include distance to stores; lower-income households may bypass their closest stores to shop at destinations with lower prices.[22] Methods like ground-truthing or robust spatial analysis that go beyond shop proximity are needed to fully understand the role of dollar stores in the American diet.[21,23] In addition, while this study only explored food expenditures in dollar stores, future studies should assess the types of foods being purchased and healthfulness of those foods through indicators such as the Healthy Eating Index. Lastly, our study reveals strong regional differences in food purchases in dollar stores, but is not well-positioned to explain those differences.

Public Health Implications

The increasing market share of dollar stores, especially in rural areas, calls for more attention to dollar stores and their role as food retailers. As dollar stores become a major source of food-at-home purchases for rural communities, understanding the quality of the foods they offer is warranted. AJPH

ABOUT THE AUTHORS

Wenhui Feng is with the Department of Public Health and Community Medicine, Tufts University, Boston, MA. Elina T. Page is with the Economic Research Service, US Department of Agriculture, Washington, DC. Sean B. Cash is with the Friedman School of Nutrition Science and Policy, Tufts University.

CORRESPONDENCE

Correspondence should be sent to Wenhui Feng, 136 Harrison Ave, Boston, MA 02111 (e-mail: wenhui.feng@tufts.edu). Reprints can be ordered at https://ajph.org by clicking the "Reprints" link.

PUBLICATION INFORMATION

Full Citation: Feng W, Page ET, Cash SB. Dollar stores and food access for rural households in the United States, 2008–2020. *Am J Public Health*. 2023;113(3):331–336.

Acceptance Date: November 23, 2022.

DOI: https://doi.org/10.2105/AJPH.2022.307193

CONTRIBUTORS

W. Feng led the study. All authors contributed to the study design, analysis, and drafting the article. All authors read and approved the final article.

ACKNOWLEDGMENTS

This study was supported in part by US Department of Agriculture (USDA) Cooperative Agreement (58-4000-0-0021) and Tufts University Springboard award (M530868).

The authors would like to thank Bangyao Sun and Divya Saravana for assisting with the analysis, and Hailey Fromkin for editorial assistance.

Note. The findings and conclusions in this publication are those of the authors and should not be construed to represent any official USDA or US government determination or policy. The analysis, findings, and conclusions expressed in this publication also should not be attributed to Information Resources Inc.

CONFLICTS OF INTEREST

No authors have conflicts of interest to report.

HUMAN PARTICIPANT PROTECTION

The Tufts Social, Behavioral, and Educational Research institutional review board reviewed the protocol and deemed this study is not research involving human participants.

REFERENCES

1. Stevens A, Cho C, Cakir M, Kong X, Boland MA. The food retail landscape across rural America. US Department of Agriculture. 2021. Available at: http://www.ers.usda.gov/publications/pub-details/?pubid=101355. Accessed May 23, 2022.
2. Caspi CE, Pelletier JE, Harnack L, Erickson DJ, Laska MN. Differences in healthy food supply and stocking practices between small grocery stores, gas-marts, pharmacies and dollar stores. *Public Health Nutr*. 2016;19(3):540–547. https://doi.org/10.1017/S1368980015002724
3. MacGillis A. The true cost of dollar stores. *The New Yorker*. June 29, 2020. Available at: https://www.newyorker.com/magazine/2020/07/06/the-true-cost-of-dollar-stores. Accessed October 28, 2022.
4. Powell LM, Slater S, Mirtcheva D, Bao Y, Chaloupka FJ. Food store availability and neighborhood characteristics in the United States. *Prev Med*. 2007;44(3):189–195. https://doi.org/10.1016/j.ypmed.2006.08.008
5. Rhone A, Ploeg MV, Williams R, Breneman V. Understanding low-income and low-access census tracts across the nation: subnational and subpopulation estimates of access to healthy food. US Department of Agriculture. 2019. Available at: http://www.ers.usda.gov/publications/pub-details/?pubid=93140. Accessed May 23, 2022.
6. Morland K, Diez Roux AV, Wing S. Supermarkets, other food stores, and obesity: the Atherosclerosis Risk in Communities Study. *Am J Prev Med*. 2006;30(4):333–339. https://doi.org/10.1016/j.amepre.2005.11.003
7. Powell LM, Auld MC, Chaloupka FJ, O'Malley PM, Johnston LD. Associations between access to food stores and adolescent body mass index. *Am J Prev Med*. 2007;33(4, suppl):S301–S307. https://doi.org/10.1016/j.amepre.2007.07.007
8. Li Y, Luo M, Wu X, Xiao Q, Luo J, Jia P. Grocery store access and childhood obesity: a systematic review and meta-analysis. *Obes Rev*. 2021;22(suppl 1):e12945. https://doi.org/10.1111/obr.12945
9. Allcott H, Diamond R, Dubé JP, Handbury J, Rahkovsky I, Schnell M. Food deserts and the causes of nutritional inequality. *Q J Econ*. 2019;134(4):1793–1844. https://doi.org/10.1093/qje/qjz015
10. Trivedi T, Liu J, Probst J, Merchant A, Jhones S, Martin AB. Obesity and obesity-related behaviors among rural and urban adults in the USA. *Rural Remote Health*. 2015;15(4):3267. https://doi.org/10.22605/RRH3267
11. US Department of Agriculture, Economic Research Service. Rural–urban commuting area codes. August 17, 2020. Available at: https://www.ers.usda.gov/data-products/rural-urban-commuting-area-codes.aspx. Accessed April 26, 2022.
12. Shoulberg W. Dollar stores, big lots, off-pricers will open thousands of stores in 2022. *Forbes*. January 16, 2022. Available at: https://www.forbes.com/sites/warrenshoulberg/2022/01/16/dollar-stores-big-lots-off-pricers-will-open-thousands-of-stores-in-2022. Accessed May 23, 2022.
13. Morris F. How Dollar General is transforming rural America. *NPR*. December 11, 2017. Available at: https://www.npr.org/2017/12/11/569815331/loving-and-hating-dollar-general-in-rural-america. Accessed May 23, 2022.
14. Troy M. Dollar General adding produce to 10,000 stores. *Progressive Grocer*. July 1, 2021. Available at: https://progressivegrocer.com/dollar-general-adding-produce-10000-stores. Accessed May 23, 2022.
15. Center for Science in the Public Interest. The rise of dollar stores: how the proliferation of discount stores may limit healthy food access. 2020. Available at: https://cspinet.org/sites/default/files/attachment/Dollar%20Store%20Fact%20Sheet.pdf. Accessed February 13, 2020.
16. Mitchell S, Donahue M. Report: dollar stores are targeting struggling urban neighborhoods and small towns. One community is showing how to fight back. Institute for Local Self-Reliance. 2018. Available at: https://ilsr.org/dollar-stores-target-cities-towns-one-fights-back. Accessed October 25, 2022.

17. McCarthy J, Minovi D, Singleton CR. Local measures to curb dollar store growth: a policy scan. *Nutrients.* 2022;14(15):3092. https://doi.org/10.3390/nu14153092

18. Chenarides L, Cho C, Nayga RM, Thomsen MR. Dollar stores and food deserts. *Appl Geogr.* 2021;134:102497. https://doi.org/10.1016/j.apgeog.2021.102497

19. Bitto EA, Morton LW, Oakland MJ, Sand M. Grocery store access patterns in rural food deserts. *J Study Food Soc.* 2003;6(2):35–48. https://doi.org/10.2752/152897903786769616

20. Grandjean AC. Dietary intake data collection: challenges and limitations. *Nutr Rev.* 2012;70(suppl 2):S101–S104. https://doi.org/10.1111/j.1753-4887.2012.00545.x

21. Sharkey JR. Measuring potential access to food stores and food-service places in rural areas in the U.S. *Am J Prev Med.* 2009;36(4, suppl):S151–S155. https://doi.org/10.1016/j.amepre.2009.01.004

22. LeDoux TF, Vojnovic I. Going outside the neighborhood: the shopping patterns and adaptations of disadvantaged consumers living in the lower eastside neighborhoods of Detroit, Michigan. *Health Place.* 2013;19:1–14. https://doi.org/10.1016/j.healthplace.2012.09.010

23. Shannon J, Reese AM, Ghosh D, Widener MJ, Block DR. More than mapping: improving methods for studying the geographies of food access. *Am J Public Health.* 2021;111(8):1418–1422. https://doi.org/10.2105/AJPH.2021.306339

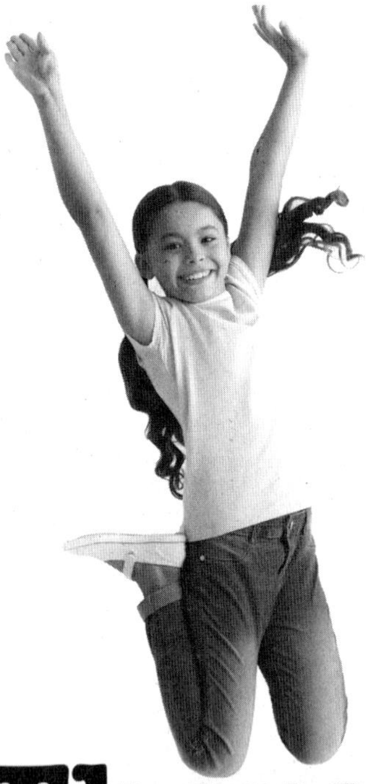

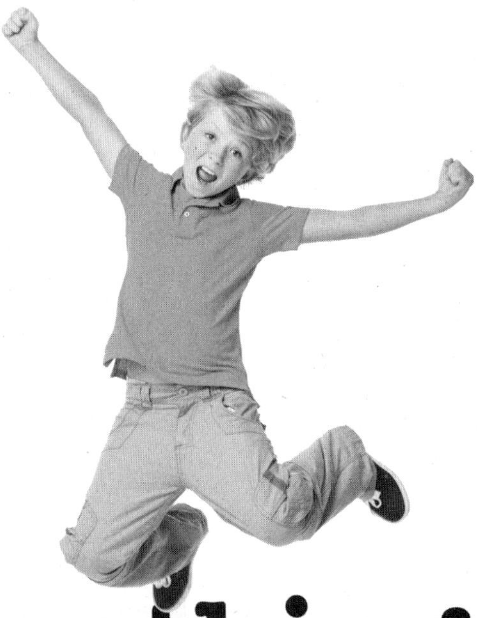

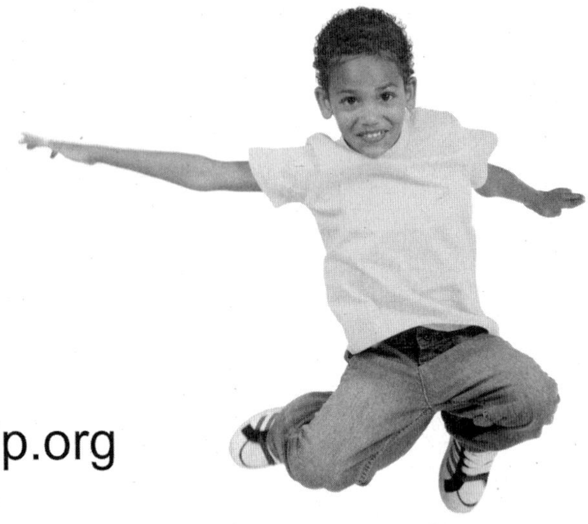

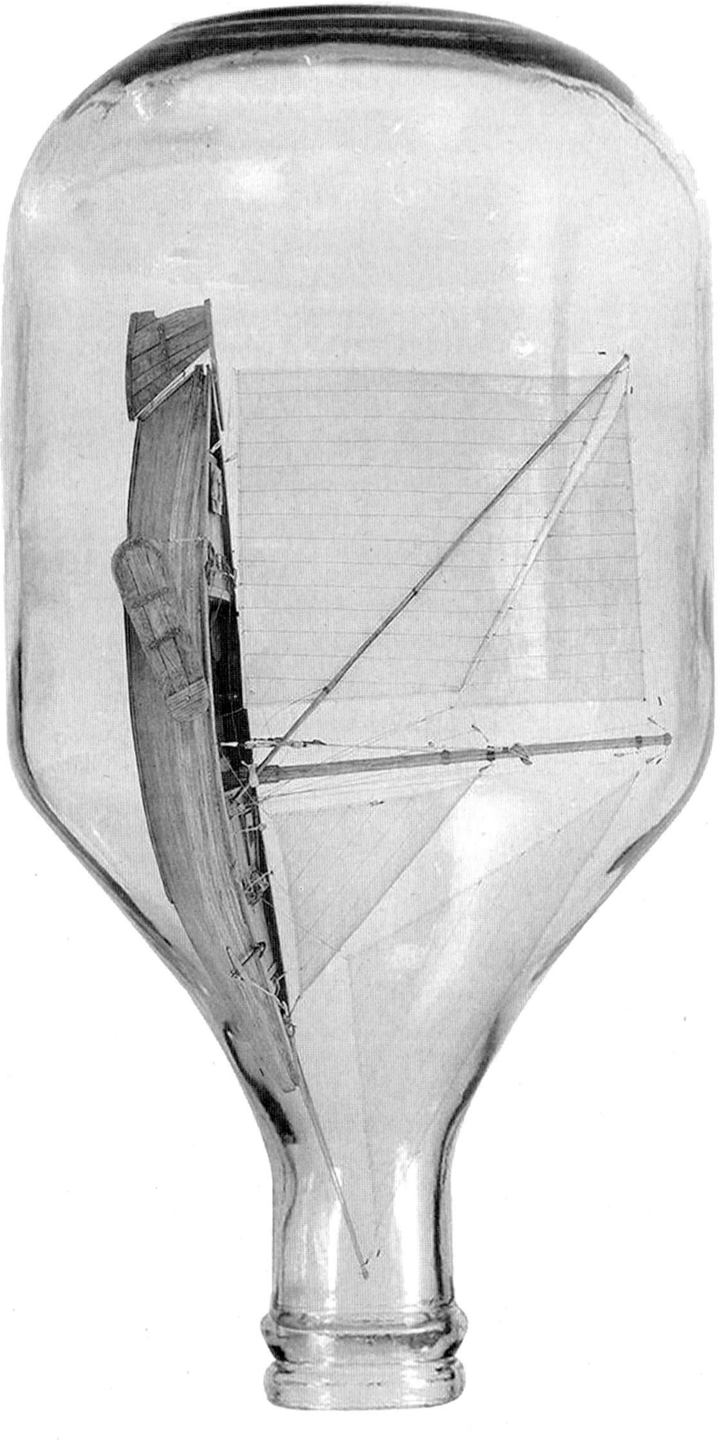

WATER
WHAT IS IT WORTH TO YOU?

Our aging water and wastewater systems are at risk.

BE AWARE
Know your water and wastewater service providers.

BE PREPARED
Store at least 3 gallons of water per family member.

SHOW YOU CARE
Support water system upgrades.

EPA

In partnership with your local water utilities.

Learn more at **water.epa.gov**

APHA Public Health Buyer's Guide

Products, services, education programs, and resources focused on furthering the work of public health professionals.

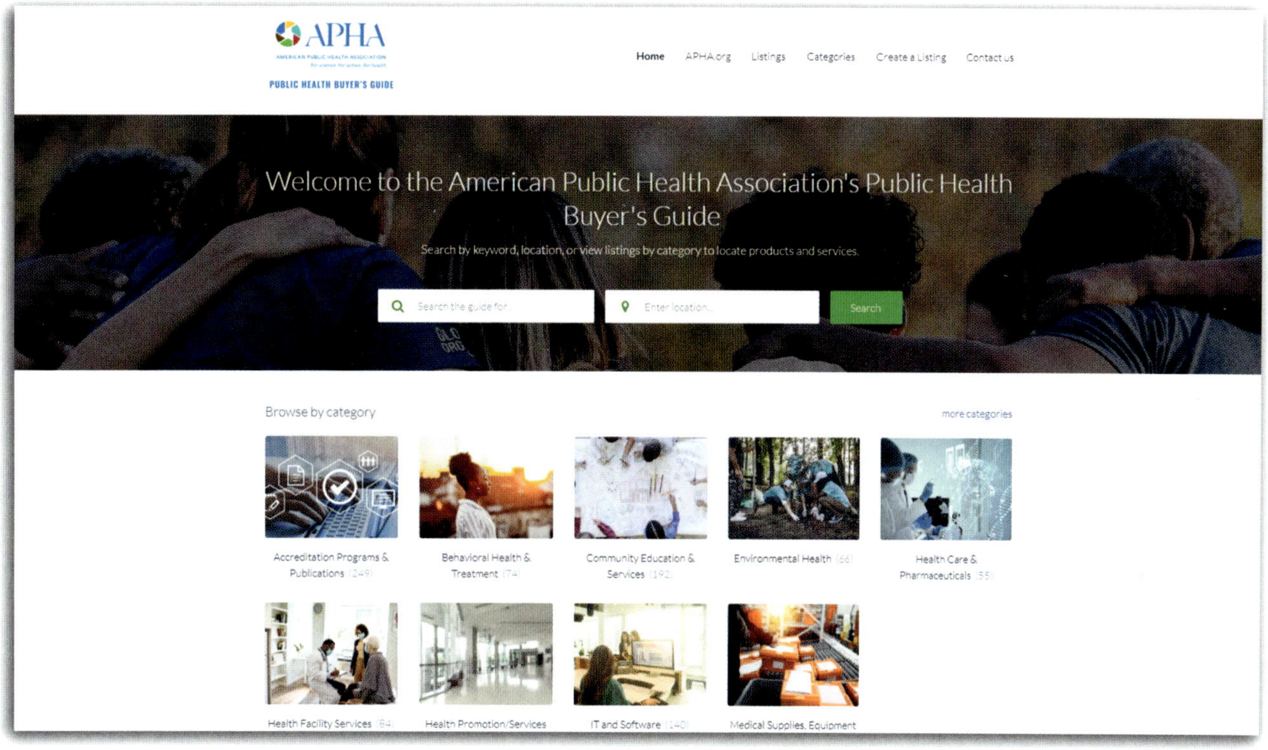

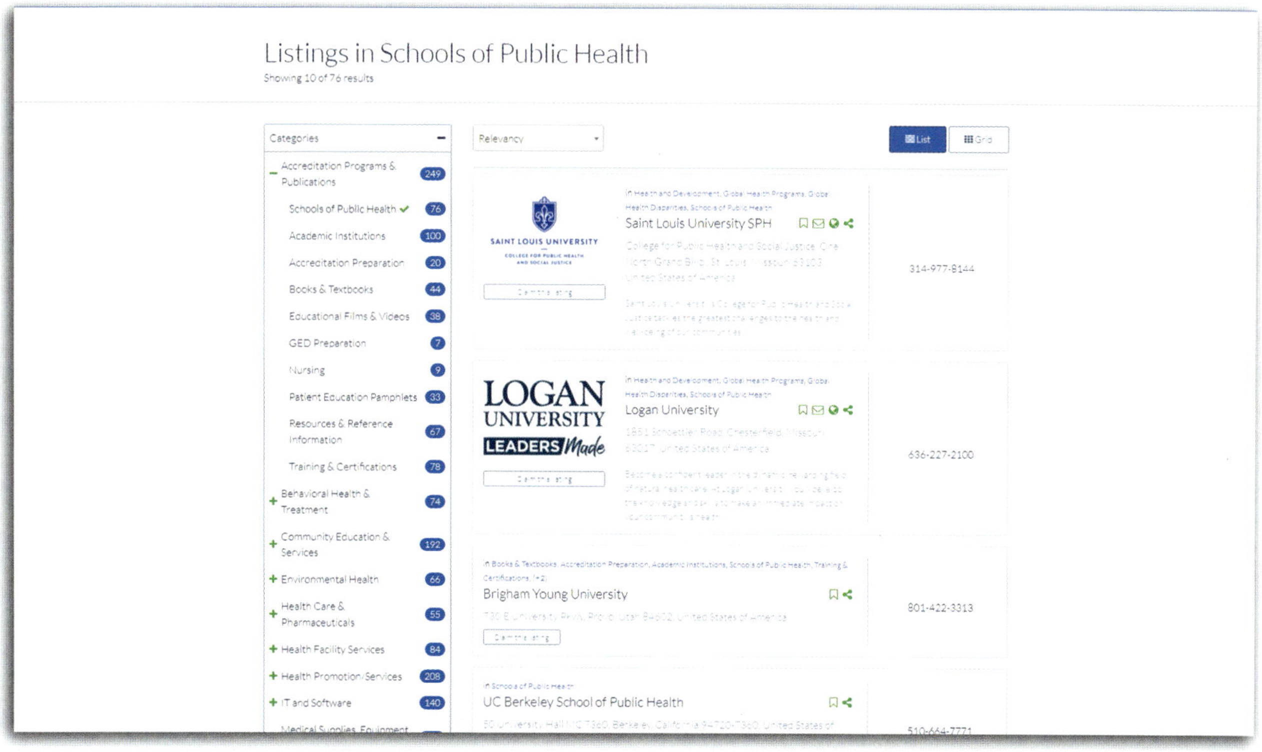

APHABuyersGuide.com

APHA
AMERICAN PUBLIC HEALTH ASSOCIATION
For science. For action. For health.